For Joe

Stroke: A Long, Challenging Journey

A True Story

wishing you good health!

by
Peter Frost

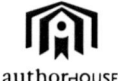
Bloomington, IN   Milton Keynes, UK
authorHOUSE®

AuthorHouse™
1663 Liberty Drive, Suite 200
Bloomington, IN 47403
www.authorhouse.com
Phone: 1-800-839-8640

AuthorHouse™ *UK Ltd.*
500 Avebury Boulevard
Central Milton Keynes, MK9 2BE
www.authorhouse.co.uk
Phone: 08001974150

This book is a work of non-fiction. Unless otherwise noted, the author and the publisher make no explicit guarantees as to the accuracy of the information contained in this book and in some cases, names of people and places have been altered to protect their privacy.

© 2006 Peter Frost. All rights reserved.

No part of this book may be reproduced, stored in a retrieval system, or transmitted by any means without the written permission of the author.

First published by AuthorHouse 12/14/2006

ISBN: 978-1-4259-7863-1 (sc)

Library of Congress Control Number: 2006910053

Printed in the United States of America
Bloomington, Indiana

This book is printed on acid-free paper.

Set in 14 pt font for visually impaired.

To my wife and best friend, Hélène, with so many thanks and much appreciation for her love, support, care and enduring patience during my recovery efforts and the assembly of this book and thanks to our three boys, for always making me proud.

With all my love,

PF

Contents

Acknowledgements   xi
Prologue   xiii

Section One – The Early Years

Chapter 1:	All You Need Is Love	3
Chapter 2:	The Squeeky Wheel Gets The Oil	9
Chapter 3:	Laughs In Mixed Company	15
Chapter 4:	A Mind Of My Own	17
Chapter 5:	Man And His World	21
Chapter 6:	Magical Playground	23
Chapter 7:	Fires, Fires And Bigger Fires	25
Chapter 8:	Rock Concerts	28
Chapter 9:	Nothing's Going To Change My World	31
Chapter 10:	Youth Hostels	33
Chapter 11:	A Wonderful New Life	37
Chapter 12:	The Mod Squad	41
Chapter 13:	Close Call	43
Chapter 14:	The Guinea Pig	47
Chapter 15:	Life Goes On	49
Chapter 16:	Madoc Pop Festival	51

Section Two – Moving On

Chapter 1:	Sports, Games And More Games	57
Chapter 2:	Newfoundlanders, Pitchers And Good Competition	59
Chapter 3:	Onward And Upward	63
Chapter 4:	Lake Placid 1980 Winter Olympic Games	65
Chapter 5:	Corporate Upheaval	70

Section Three – No Reply

Chapter 1:	I've Just Seen A Face	77
Chapter 2:	Day-to-Day Life	80
Chapter 3:	Loud Mouth Louie's	88

Section Four – If Only I Had Known

Chapter 1:	I Should Have Known Better	93
Chapter 2:	Code Blue	97
Chapter 3:	Criti-Call	106
Chapter 4:	What In The World Is S.A.R.S.?	108

Section Five – A New Life

Chapter 1:	Here, There and Everywhere	117
Chapter 2:	Wedding Planning	128
Chapter 3:	Here Comes the Bride	136
Chapter 4:	Special People	141
Chapter 5:	Chronology of my Rebirth	147
Chapter 6:	A Bump in the Road	150
Chapter 7:	Rehabilitation	154

Section Six – Reconstruction (The People In My Life)

Chapter 1:	People in Your Life	161
Chapter 2:	Routines	163
Chapter 3:	Two Special Angels	168
Chapter 4:	Special Words About and for Caregivers	171
Chapter 5:	It's Only Love	172
Chapter 6:	Neighbours From Heaven	178
Chapter 7:	The GFCI From Hell	182
Chapter 8:	All Together Now	184
Chapter 9:	Fun and Games Around Our Court	186
Chapter 10:	With a Little Help From Our Friends	188
Chapter 11:	Those Were The Days	193

Section Seven – Life Goes On

Chapter 1:	Get Ready, I'm Coming	201
Chapter 2:	The Creek	207
Chapter 3:	The Golf Cart	209
Chapter 4:	The ATM	211
Chapter 5:	The Clubs	213
Chapter 6:	The Pool Table	215
Chapter 7:	The Dryer	218
Chapter 8:	The Bus Stop	220
Chapter 9:	The Taxi	221
Chapter 10:	The Lawn Mower	223

Section Eight – Things I've Tried

Chapter 1:	The Eagles' Farewell Concert and Other Diversions	229
Chapter 2:	My Quest Continues	236
Chapter 3:	The Basic Principles Behind TCM	254
Chapter 4:	I'll Try Anything Once	258
Chapter 5:	Not a Quitter	269
Chapter 6:	A New Life…Fore!	271
Chapter 7:	My Recovery Hobby: And Here They Are… The Beatles	273
Chapter 8:	Support Groups	276

Section Nine – A Few Things You Should Know

Chapter 1:	High Blood Pressure and What It Can Do To You	283
Chapter 2:	Stroke, Complex Central Pain Syndrome and Thalamic Pain Syndrome	286
Chapter 3:	Complex Regional Pain Syndrome	296
Chapter 4:	Sleep Apnea and Hypertension	298
Chapter 5:	Fish Oil and the Brain	321

Section Ten – Let Me Say This About That

Chapter 1:	Customer Service Excellence	329
Chapter 2:	My Customer Service Experience	344
Chapter 3:	Slow Down	347

Section Eleven – From Me To You

Chapter 1:	Perseverance is the Best Medicine	353
Chapter 2:	A Brain Teaser	356
Chapter 3:	A Positive Attitude	357
Chapter 4:	Become Informed	358
Chapter 5:	Don't Sweat the Small Stuff	361
Epilogue		362

Appendix

A Stroke Survivor's Journal - How I Feel   369

ACKNOWLEDGEMENTS

I wish to express my thanks to my friends and loved ones for their unending support and encouragement.

Also, I want to thank my Taoist Tai Chi friends: my co-participant and assistant instructor Helen Crowe, for her critique of some of this book and for sharing her creative writing skills with me; my friends and co-participants, Andy and Drew, for allowing me to interview them and for sharing their insight and experiences.

Thanks are certainly due to my many personal support workers, including Leanne, Debbie, Susan, Tom, Nicole, Patricia, Jasmine and others who have filled in for each other from time to time – thank you so much for always listening and for offering your opinions, whether or not I asked for them!

I also wish to convey a special thank you to a dear friend and supporter, Kelly Ekman, for staying up most of the night at one of our Health Recovery weeks to read over some of my latest words in my creation of this book and for her honest and encouraging reaction and support.

Special thanks go to our friend Alena Moravcova, who graciously permitted me to use the cover photo, which was taken during her last trip to Barbados with my best friend, Dave, just months before his passing; to our son Tyler, for the beautiful drawings he provided for this book; and to our son Paul, for the heartfelt poem he contributed.

When I was a child, I felt immortal.
When I was a teenager, I felt invincible.
Since my illness, I feel vulnerable.

Author Unknown

PROLOGUE

At first glance, Peter, a 53 year-old professional, has been living a fairly simple, busy, but predictable life. With his wife and three sons, he lives in a modest back-split just outside Toronto. However, for Peter, this ordinary life is the result of an extraordinary journey. This is his story.

I am writing this book for a few reasons, not the least of which is that I have wanted to write a book for a few years. I now find myself in a perfect situation and with lots of time to do so. In fact, I have expanded my goal to try to provide assistance to other stroke survivors by sharing some personal experiences and researched data that hopefully will help them understand the trauma that a stroke survivor goes through. In addition, it was my initial hope that this little project would provide me with some therapeutic assistance for my brain, assistance further to what my wonderful occupational therapist, Jennifer, at Bridgepoint Health had provided.

As you read on, you will learn that I have had two strokes and, in fact, that I am simply just lucky to be alive. I want to share my journey because it is just that, a journey with many curves, surprises and disappointments and with many challenges that need to be overcome. I am so lucky to have my wife and my children by my side. They have all been so supportive and helpful throughout my ordeal. As well, our two year old Golden Retriever, Cooper (for my re*cooper*ation) has been extremely therapeutic for me. I love them all to bits and honestly, I don't know what I would have done without them.

I need to, once again, thank my wife for all the support and the tenuous editing we have done together in writing this book. We were fortunate enough to be able to pool our resources and our talents and work together to create this project. Prior to my illness, my wife was an administrative assistant in a school board and she worked with and for some amazing people. Oh, man! We had some nice and very special brunches, lunches and dinners with many of them. We joined them to enjoy those occasions with the love of God and the support of some very special professionals. Thank you Madeleine, André, Carole, Daniel and all the others who contributed to make those times so special.

I have just been talking to Paul, my musically talented, adventurous and globetrotting 25 year old stepson, and have asked him to compose a special song or poem as a theme for my adventure. Based on what we have already seen him do for our wedding two years ago, I know we can expect something special from him. Thanks, Paul! In fact, I have enclosed Paul's poem for your reading pleasure. You will find it at the end of Section Six, Chapter 5.

I have asked my artistically talented 20 year old son, Tyler, to create some art work for this book. All his life, he has displayed a natural artistic talent that never ceases to amaze and impress me, or anyone else, for that matter! Please review some of his work on the adjacent pages. Anytime someone comes over to visit, they always marvel at the incredible drawings on the walls of his room. He has so much promise and I am sure he is going somewhere with his natural ability. We are so proud!

My 15 year old son, Corey, has thankfully more than done his part for us and himself in the past couple of years, achieving straight A's or equivalent consistently throughout his first 10 years of schooling and rarely missing a day or being late for a class. I thank you for that, Corey. I can't tell you enough how much your conscientiousness allows an ailing parent to be able to focus on other things like healing and recovery that are crucial and so important and just won't take care of themselves. The university years are exciting ones facing a sixteen year old and, for Corey, they are now just around the corner. I am sure he just can't wait.

So, imagine for a minute the impact of sailing, headfirst, through your car windshield in a 110 km/h collision. The trauma to your brain has changed your life forever. You have lost the use of one or both sides of your body. You are instantly unable to make others understand what you are saying, and, even worse, you cannot understand what they are saying. Imagine never being able to return to your career or take care of your family again.

Now, imagine that you never left your living room and never had that car accident. Even so, in one single moment, losses such as these, the result of devastating brain trauma, are now defining your entire existence. That is stroke!

Close to three-quarters of a million people, almost one-quarter of a million of working age or younger (even children and infants), experience stroke each year in the United States alone, where stroke is the Number One cause of long-term disability among adults. Stroke is the second leading cause of death in the entire world, killing 4.6 million people annually.

Stroke is physically, mentally, emotionally, spiritually, socially, and economically debilitating. While there are varying risk factors, stroke can happen to anyone, regardless of age, race, socioeconomic status, or even general health.

It is vital for everyone to be alerted to this threat: how to recognize the symptoms of stroke and how one can best minimize chances of being killed or severely disabled by stroke. I want to let the world know the incredible toll that stroke takes on survivors, their families, medicine and society.

I have decided to write this book in order to share my experiences with you and with others who may also have had a stroke. Hopefully, the knowledge I have gained and the information we have collected over the past three and a half years, which I am now attempting to share, will benefit others who may be susceptible to or who may have experienced the same tragic event. For those of you who are or have been in my situation, hopefully my story will reassure you that you are not alone and that what you are feeling, be it physical or emotional, is absolutely predictable and is just a phase in the entire healing process. You will improve and get better with determination and perseverance. I hope my thoughts and the feelings I have expressed are helpful in getting you through this.

As well, in this writing, I am trying to settle my damaged brain and provide a clear and unique perspective for others on what it is like to go through a catastrophe such as this in order that they may benefit from someone else's experience. My wonderful wife has given me reason to carry on. So have our Golden Retriever and our sons. What is important to understand is that everything in such a life is surreal and that my head has a constant buzz and pressure that just won't quit. There are moments when clear thinking just doesn't happen and depression takes over all concentration and logical thinking.

I am extremely grateful to the very special people in my stroke rehab and support groups and my Taoist Tai Chi Health Recovery classes for their friendship and support throughout my adventure. My friends, I write this book for you! Thank you for the feedback, the love and the encouragement. Because of you, I am blessed and my future is promising!

I also must tell you that I never saw this brain attack coming at all. I am writing this story to inform others about what I went through (and am still going through) so that they can be prepared in the event that they must also face this type of situation. With a bit of luck and a great deal of determination, some of these ideas may help them find a way to hopefully avoid or overcome such a calamity and rebuild their own neurological abilities and regain their former functionality. I only wish someone had forewarned me at the time. While some of the signs were there, I was not educated enough on this subject to see this disaster coming and possibly prevent it from taking over my life. Also, I am taking this opportunity to provide some education, albeit from my perspective and within the scope of my limited knowledge and experience. Almost every day, we are seeing something about the warning signs of stroke either on TV or in advertisements. Well, I can tell you that these warning signs are just a little too late. The ads I have seen on TV and in brochures in hospitals tell of signs of the onset of stroke, signs such as dizziness, headaches, blurred vision, etc. Well, if you are experiencing any or most of these symptoms, it is probably too late and you have already had a stroke. Does it mean you should not seek immediate attention? Absolutely not! It means you should call 9-1-1 and go to the emergency department at the nearest hospital right away. It absolutely will mean the difference between saving your life or not and preventing permanent and painful disability.

The point I am trying to make is that these warning signs simply mean that you are about to have or have already had a stroke. In some cases, this means that you may already have had some serious brain damage resulting in permanent paralysis and/or other damage. I believe that what is required is better education on how to take proper care of yourself and prevent such a disaster. This involves having your blood pressure checked regularly by your family physician and, in the event it is too high, religiously taking the blood pressure medication your doctor prescribes. Of course, also of importance are proper exercise, a good diet, alcohol only in moderation, no smoking and a balanced lifestyle including a good work ethic and a moderate stress level. I remind you here that I am certainly no physician, nor am I qualified to give specific advice in this highly specialized and critical area; but I am now experienced and living the results and simply know what I wish I had done to prevent these horrible consequences. You are about to read about my nightmare, my life and near death, including the life-impacting consequences that I cry and think about much of the time. I heartily recommend that you immediately do some follow-up and research into how something like this can happen to you whether you are 25 (less likely but it happens), 49 (my category) or 60 or older (highest percentage).

The way I see it, the worst thing you can do to yourself is to not monitor or pay proper attention to your blood pressure. Of course, I am not a doctor, nor am I qualified or licensed to give advice or recommendations except maybe to tell you to see your family physician regularly before something like this strikes you. Let me tell you, this disastrous medical affliction can sneak up on you without warning and your life may be significantly changed before you know it. Life as you knew it can be over. Please understand that this book is in no way intended to represent any official medical authority, but rather it is simply a depiction of my life and the events I experienced prior to, during and since my strokes.

I truly hope that, in reading my story, you are able to understand this potential threat better than I did and thereby avoid such devastation to your life and your body. Trust me, the therapies and treatments are no fun and there are no guarantees. Then there's the damned medicine. At this time, I am required to take about 24 pills per day, including Altace, Labetalol, Norvasc and Hydrochlorothiazide to keep my blood pressure under control and Ranitidine to protect my stomach from all these medicines. In addition, I take Detrol for my urinary tract, Calcium, Baclofen, a muscle relaxant, Temazepam, to help me sleep at night and Gabapentin for dizziness. I also take some over-the-counter medications including Vitamin B-Complex (for nerve regeneration), cranberry tablets, Senokot, Soflax and Lactulose. I could open my own pharmacy, don't you think? Hélène has to go to the pharmacy an average of twice a week as we frequently run out of something critical. We have medical insurance for most of the essential prescriptions; however this does not quite cover all of the needs, as dispensing fees are not covered.

As you progress through this book, you will learn that one of the worst effects of my stroke was the brain damage I was left with as a result of my first brain attack, resulting in a short-term memory deficit. I have had to learn to manage this problem by writing things down as they come to mind. I also purchased a Palm Pilot which allows me to take notes, create documents and files, check my calendar and basically just keep track of my life, activities and appointments. If I don't keep some form of record, I will simply forget what it was I needed or wanted to do or was thinking about, causing me intense frustration. I am extremely dizzy most of the time and it feels like there is a hive of angry bees buzzing inside my head. If you can try to imagine this, the dizziness is with me 24/7 and there is no relief or escape. Each waking moment is the same. The more I think and concentrate, the more the buzzing intensifies. Augghh! I need rescuing! With no exaggeration, help me please! And oh yes, it does hurt! The pressure is unrelenting!

Since I have been attempting to write this book, I have been extremely motivated to jot hundreds of ideas down as each day goes by. Through this book, it is my intention to try to share with you just how this experience feels and how incredibly frustrating it is to not be taken seriously when your life consists of one continuing and terribly complex event after the other.

For example, I went through several months of repeated urinary tract infections that just didn't seem to want to go away. I suffered a series of painful symptoms with which I had become too familiar. I took a medication for this and usually after three to five days, I eventually felt a little better, but not necessarily 100%. This was usually around the time that I had taken my last pill in the latest bottle of medicine. Of course, because I was not quite feeling 100% when I took the last pill and because I had not yet been given the "all clear" with a urine test, the next thing I knew the full rampage of the infection was back again. I have learned somewhat how my own body works and, in this situation, with a bladder infection and how terrible it makes me feel, I was literally "scared to death" of any possibility of a reoccurrence.

If you have ever had the occasion to be "scared to death" of something, let me tell you that many thoughts can and do come to mind! I certainly don't like bladder infections!

I am not an expert writer by any means, although I am pretty good with grammar and spelling, I guess due to my achievements in high school and some post-secondary education. You will find out later that this skill likely contributed to my stroke and nearly resulted in my death, but more on that later. I think I am compelled to write this book about my life because technically, I should be dead! I did die! I was a "Code Blue" in the hospital! Luckily, I have been granted the good fortune to live on. To live on in this faulty shell, but I am loved and I have a purpose. Damn, I am even determined that I will walk and even play guitar again. I would like to help others too. I would like some of those others to walk with me. Also, I would like those of you who have had the good fortune to have avoided this awful disaster so far to take care of yourselves, get your blood pressure checked and make sure you don't have one of these nightmares. It is not fun! It hurts. Be forewarned!

After all, there is no guarantee that you'll get a second chance, if this happens to you, because you just may not. Some of us are luckier than others, I guess.

So this is my story. This is also my life. Some people would call what has happened to me a tragedy. I am choosing to look at it as an opportunity. I hope you find this book informative and entertaining.

P.F.

P.S. A friend of ours recently told me of a problem she is having with controlling her blood pressure. Another friend also called us recently to tell us she was experiencing symptoms similar to those I had gone through as I was about to have my stroke. Well, Martina and Elise, a free copy of my book is on its way to you with our love and best wishes. Hélène and I are so worried about you both, because we are living the hell that you could possibly also go through. Anything you can do is worth doing to make sure nothing awful like this ever happens to you. Your friends and family do love you but might not or do not always get around to saying so until it's too late! Gosh, I think someone should write a book about this!

SECTION ONE – THE EARLY YEARS

CHAPTER 1: ALL YOU NEED IS LOVE

It has become a goal of mine to retrace my early years and to share my memories and experiences with my friends and acquaintances from that time of my life, as well as with anyone else who wants to listen. I have found this exercise to be extremely therapeutic, considering my brain damage and subsequent short-term memory deficit. I also find that recapturing these times is a lot like actually reliving my youth, which all of a sudden seems to have flown by so quickly. I do have a strong urge to remember these times as well as relive and even go back to them. My brain churns all the time, generating new ideas, concepts and schemes. I daydream 24/7 and I am constantly regenerating my thoughts and thinking about the many good times I had in my youth. Ask my wife. This brain activity keeps us both hopping. You should see our calendar of daily and weekly appointments and activities! There isn't a day that goes by that we don't have some type of event, whether it's Tai Chi, our support group, a doctor's appointment, physiotherapy, a session with my personal trainer, homecare or whatever. We never stop or have a dull moment!

It's interesting to note that one side effect of my strokes has been that I seem to have fast-tracked and forgotten many of the years of my pre-stroke life. Even though I know I'm 53, I feel like I should only be about 35 years old or less, in spite of my current disability and my physical and mental challenges. With my memory lapses, it's as though my life is on videotape and someone has cut out a few feet of tape every so often throughout the ongoing saga and adventures of my life.

I lived in Montréal with my Mom and Dad from the time I was born until I was 18 when we moved to Ontario. My brother and sister were always somewhere in the family picture, doing their thing at their respective ages. I believe they were happy kids also, doing lots of younger sister and brother stuff in their own age groups with their little gangs of friends. Being three and five years older than them respectively, I was simply doing older brother things, so I guess I didn't always see them that much, except at meals, holidays and the family vacations we would go on with Mom and Dad.

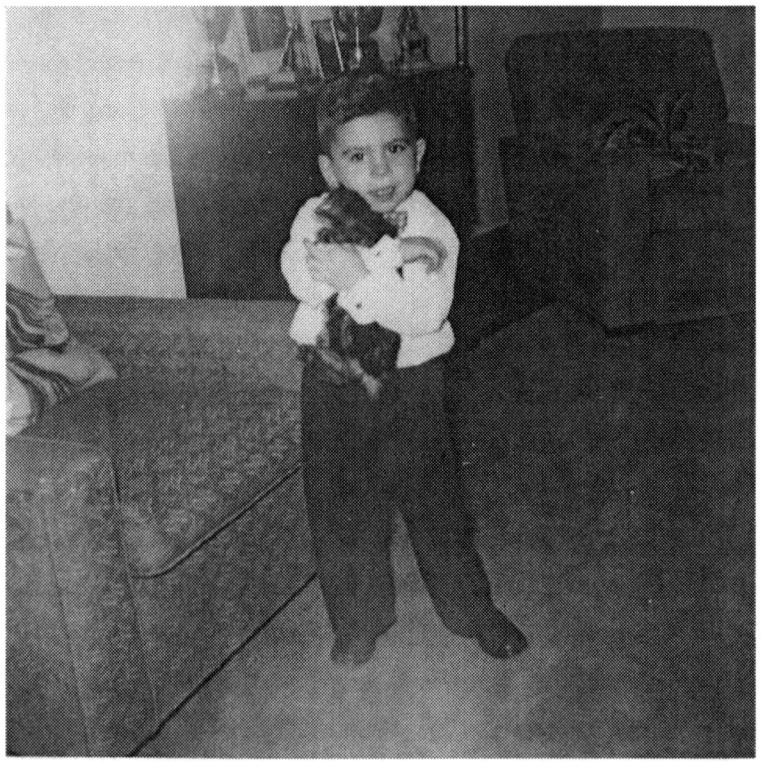

Age 3 – Cuddling my first cat, Tiggie

We were lucky kids and we were happy. We loved Mom and Dad and were proud of them. We also had the most wonderful relatives. Dad would frequently make a point of driving us to see the various aunties and uncles and cousins either at their homes in the Montréal or surrounding areas, or at their cottages if they had one. This would have been when I was somewhere between about 5 and 12 years old.

Dad also drove us fairly often to see his Mom in the Eastern Townships. We called her Dodee. She had the most magical huge old home that so clearly brings back the most amazing and precious memories. She had this stately wood frame home with wooden verandas surrounding it and cozy porches in the front and on the sides. I can still smell the many coats of aged grey and yellow painted wood. I remember some of these times like they were yesterday.

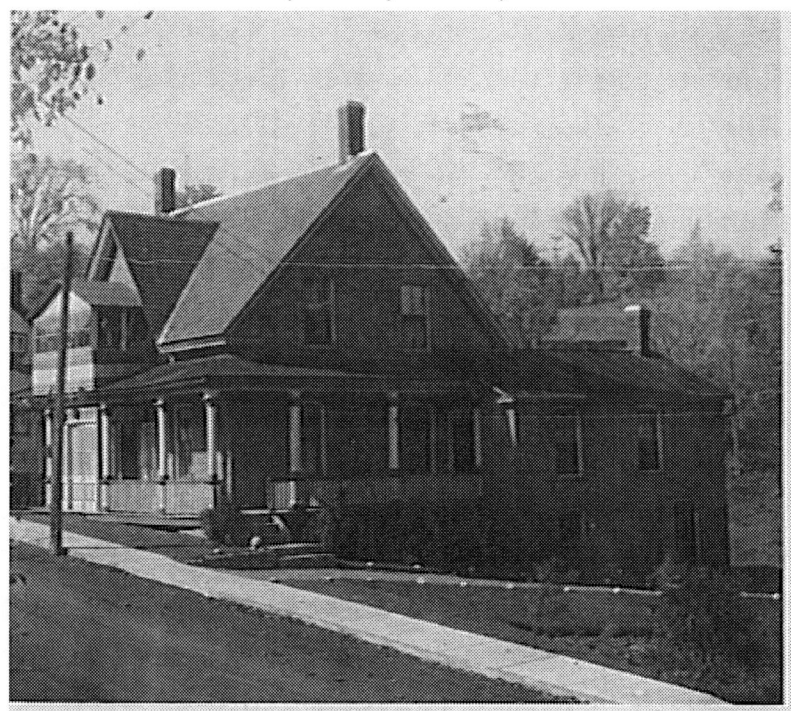

Dodee's house, ca. 1958

Occasionally, when we visited, Dad would heroically assemble torches with oily rags to burn wasp nests that had been built in the soffits earlier that year. I can also still smell the mothballs from the big old storage trunks that we would explore as kids. I remember being spooked by the old violin case that was stored behind the grand old sofa in the large, cold, dark living room. The light switches were the old, stiff, push button style.

The kitchen was always an adventure. It had a little refrigerator on legs and a wood bin with a rope-drawn vertical sliding door, usually filled with many scrap hardwood cuttings from a local furniture factory. There was also a beautiful wood stove and the most marvelous walk-in pantry where we could always find crackers, bread and fresh jams. There was also a mysterious rear alternate stairway to the upper bedroom floors.

Another magical feature we always found time to explore was the attic that was accessible from a trap door in the upstairs hallway. The access door swung down from the ceiling and Dad and I would crawl up the retractable staircase (similar to a fire escape) and into the long, dimly lit attic. It had quite a low ceiling, or so it seemed at the time, given my young age. I guess that, for a boy of 5 to 15 years old, everything is an adventure! Dad had kept his army memorabilia in his kit box and his old uniforms in his kit bag, both of which were in this room; whenever we visited, he and I would rout through the special trinkets, medals and old coins. I will always recall the time that we came across his service revolver, an old .32 that Dad actually eventually brought home as a memento or souvenir and hid in his sock drawer. I remember the day that Mom first discovered it when he actually brought it home. She immediately told him to get rid of it. I can still hear her in my mind! When Hélène and I were recently going through some of Dad's things, I came across the kit box and spent hours looking over the various papers, photos, etc. It brought back so many fond memories! I brought the kit box back to our home and will cherish it forever.

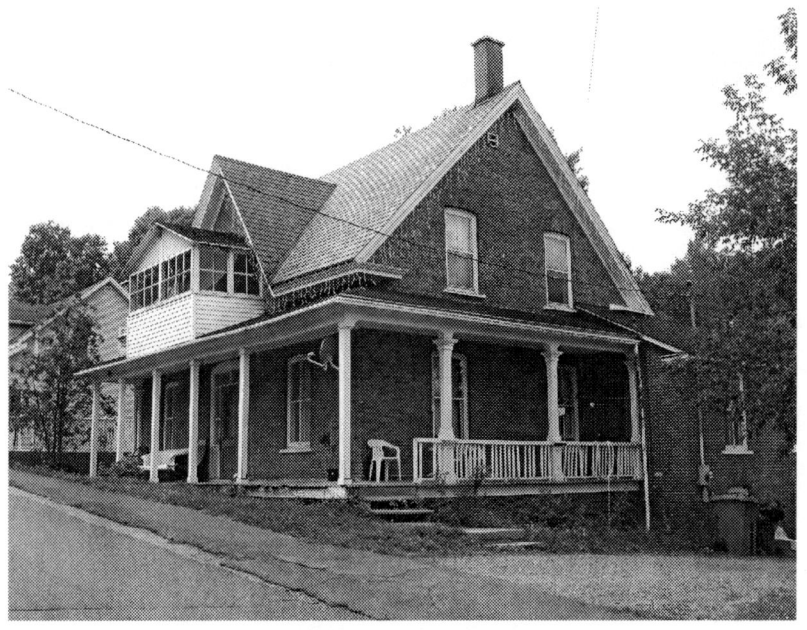

Dodee's house today

Dad would recall some of his experiences and tell me tales of the times that he and Mom had shared during, before and after the War. I remember that he told me of how he and Mom met in Aldershot, England and how they played much tennis together and went dancing often. They lived truly long, interesting and happy lives. I am so proud of and happy for them.

When I was 5, Mom and I cruised overseas to visit the relatives in the UK. We traveled abroad on two ships. The one going over was the Ivernia and the other coming back was the Saxonia. I remember fondly going to Tiny Nana's house (Mom's Mom) and spending time with my cousins Carole and Lesley who would always take me to see the trains and would take me to a shop where I grew my collection of Matchbox Dinky toys. I remember fondly playing ball in the backyard with Uncle Leo and I recall that I think I kicked the ball over the fence on him a few too many times. I was loved and we laughed a lot.

Auntie Stella, Mom's older sister, came to see us in Canada a few times and I clearly recall how she and Mom would always cry so much as they came close to the end of their visit and Auntie Stella had to pack and prepare to leave. It was always so sad when she had to leave and we would see her off at the airport. Then there was the story that Mom and Auntie Stella told me of the time they lit a Guy Fawkes Day rocket in their parents' living room, luckily avoiding setting the curtains or the house ablaze!

As you have seen frequently in my writing, kids will be kids! And Auntie Stella always said that I was her favorite. I miss Mom so much now that she is gone. As I recall these special times, I think what a shame that they are times long past and I wonder why we can't hang on to them and keep them going forever. Why do good things have to change (eyes welling up with tears for a few moments)?

I miss Mom so much now. She passed away almost two years ago at the age of 86. She and Dad played golf until they were 82 or so. When my brother and I were 36 and 42 respectively, we played a few rounds with them. Dad, I love you so much.

CHAPTER 2: THE SQUEEKY WHEEL GETS THE OIL

When I was about 10 years old, my Dad helped me build a soap box car. Damn, it was well built but frig, was it ever ugly! My friend John lived right across the street and his sister, Eva, helped him build his car and it was absolutely beautiful.

I can still see those cars today; mine was built with a 3' wide piece of heavy three-quarter inch plywood as a solid bottom base and had half-inch thick plywood sides. It was painted an ugly brown with Rez stain and John's was tastefully painted a Porsche red and was a nice looking sleek car. John called his car the *Proserpina* and mine was simply labeled *Kool Kat* with strips of white adhesive tape across the gently bent one-eighth inch plywood cowling. Dad built my car ingeniously and made it quite heavy with a low profile and a pointed nose built out of quarter inch plywood. We had used some scraps of wood that we found lying around the house because the regulations stated that there was a maximum expenditure for building each car, the only exemption being the wheels. As it turned out, Dad had designed the superior car.

After all the competitors' cars were assembled and had been painted and were ready to be pushed around the town's blocks for weeks prior to the race, we had a ball pushing them around and pretending we were actual race circuit moguls. Dad had bought me an official CFL helmet that he expected me to always wear whenever I was being pushed around in my car or racing down the steep ramp in case of a crash or roll-over. My mechanic and race partner was my neighbour, Cary, who foolishly and loyally would push me around the neighbourhood on the days prior to and including the actual race days.

Well, the time finally arrived with a full couple of weekends reserved for the races. My helmet was an ugly official green CFL helmet (I forget which team it actually was) that sort of went with my ugly brown walnut-stained car. Dad had designed a steering assembly out of a length of 1 ½" doweling, a circular cut piece of plywood as a steering wheel, all mounted on an 8" metal turntable that enabled a smooth and positive 300° radius turn on a well lubricated and precisely set series of ball bearings with a failsafe rope system to allow for emergency pull turns if necessary. He made the brake out of an appropriately shaped 2"x4" arm as a lever at the right side with a piece of rubber cut and affixed to it to ensure positive breaking action. Dad had installed four good quality 12" ball bearing wheels all around which ensured a fast, smooth ride enabled by the heavy construction. The cars were designed and built to compete in a municipal soap-box car derby being held on a 40' high scaffold and plywood ramp up at the local shopping centre parking lot. There were at least 18 entrants of 7 to 16 year olds with their cars of many styles, colors and designs.

Each driver was allowed one mechanic to assist in pushing the driver in his car up the ramp and to the starting gate as required. It was all just small time stuff but it was exciting for us and it was fun. Race day was particularly fun. The local press was there taking pictures and we were taking a few practice runs down the ramp. We were carefully supervised and monitored but I remember that on my first practice run, my mechanic allowed my car to run too far and it hit the concrete curb stone, breaking part of my steering assembly. I guess I was sort of frustrated and upset at our clumsiness and carelessness, but my Dad was right there to repair and reassemble the steering assembly and soon we were operational again.

Mine was one of the first cars pushed backward up the ramp and latched into place at the top while the starter did a "Ready, Set, Go" and set me on my way. The ride downhill was breathtaking and exciting. I nervously and firmly held the steering wheel, keeping my wheels in as straight a line as possible, picking up speed as I rolled down the quite high ramp. I made it down the ramp without incident, with a slight 'ker thump' as the front and then the back wheels hit the level pavement at the bottom of the ramp then rolled for about 20 yards, eventually coming to a slow rolling stop.

The official scorekeeper had timed each run from the launch to a finish line that was marked with chalk somewhere at the bottom of the course. Each of the drivers took a practice run and then excitedly and enviously watched the subsequent racers' trials, each of us thinking and hoping that we had had the better run. The individual times were being tallied and marked on a large cardboard score sheet somewhere at the bottom of the runway; but we weren't paying too much attention to that, meanwhile closely watching each other's runs down the ramp, catching the odd swerve and near spinout.

Finally the race had ended, all the cars having completed their runs. My mechanic, Cary, pushed me to the presentation line-up where all the cars that had successfully finished the race were assembling in front of the French guy with the microphone. Sequentially, from last to first, he called the finishers. I think there were one or two cars that had had mechanical problems and had disappointedly not been able to officially complete their runs. The Mayor of the town was there in his suit and Mayoral garb along with other counselors and elected officials. I didn't realize it at the time, being too young to understand politics, but I guess this had been a significant community event for the town.

One by one, the competitors were announced. It was an anti-climactic moment as we heard the final results sequentially announced over the P.A. system. I heard the last racers' names called then I heard my friend John's name called as the semi finalist. We were standing next to each other and yelled at each other wide-eyed, fists clenched, jumping up and down, sharing the moment and pleased at this announcement. We, of course, knew that the prizes included trophies, miscellaneous small items and even bicycles. The announcements proceeded and then there was a short pause as the announcer hesitated:

AND NOW FOR OUR GRAND PRIZE WINNER AND FIRST PLACE FINALIST: P E T E R F R O S T!

AUGH! I couldn't believe it! I had no idea! I actually had won this whole damned event. I had won a brand-new shiny red CCM bicycle and the hugest friggin' damned trophy that you could imagine.

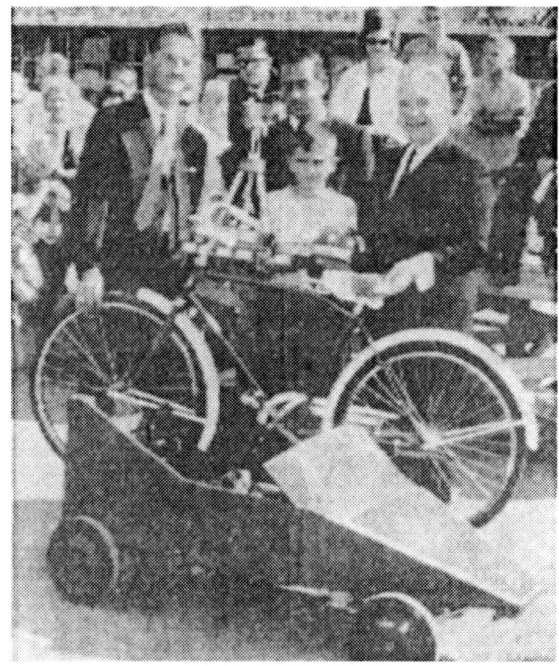

Soap box derby champion, ca. 1963

That certainly was an exciting day. Having come in second, John had also won a bicycle and he and I enjoyed our new wheels after that, riding through our neighbourhood, up to the shopping centre (where the race was and where our parents did their grocery shopping each week). Unfortunately, there was a sad ending to this story. A few weeks later, John and I rode our bikes over to Place Versailles shopping mall, a good ride and a few roads to the west of our neighbourhood, actually right beside the high school we would eventually attend. We parked our bikes in the bike rack at the front of the mall, not remembering to bring bicycle locks with us. We did naively think to come out and check on our bikes every 15 minutes or so, attempting to ensure that our bikes were not touched, taken or interfered with. Well, I think it must have been on our third or fourth check that we came out to look and sure enough, our bikes were gone, never to be seen again. What a sad, eye-opening lesson!

CHAPTER 3:   LAUGHS IN MIXED COMPANY

During my adolescence and since then, I have lived what I think has been an incredibly happy and full life. During my teens and twenties, I certainly wasn't what you would call much of a ladies' man. For the most part, I was polite in mixed company and always a gentleman. I always enjoyed hearing about some of my friends' exploits with girls and we had many laughs over some of the situations to which I was privy. From the age of 15 onward, I had what I consider to have been a particularly incredible youth and I am having a ball reliving and documenting those crazy times, especially now that I nearly died. I always lived for a good time and I did have the best of times. We were always laughing and I enjoyed and respected the wonderful friends that I played sports with and from whom I learned so much. I had so many good friends and was always doing something fun, enjoying life and making new friends.

As I said, I was not much of a ladies' man. For some reason, I was too damned shy to approach a cute girl or even start or maintain a flirtatious conversation with one. Of course, dancing was out of the question.

It wasn't that I wasn't liked or appreciated because I did make many good friends. It just seemed that some of the guys would always start to go steady before me and I seemed to be destined to be single. One of the problems was that I was always spending my time having too much fun with the guys. Many of them were pretty cool and it was way too much fun to be hanging out or playing sports or making music with them. At around age 17, we had started drinking, mostly beer. Because I had grown a moustache at around age fifteen, I could usually pass for the legal drinking age (I think 19 back then) and could easily get into the bars and clubs at a rather young age, which I thought was pretty convenient at the time.

CHAPTER 4:   A MIND OF MY OWN

Youth has its trials and tribulations. The definition of youth can also be a matter of perspective. In this situation, it all amounted to age, maturity, growing up and who thought he/she was in charge. One Saturday morning, when I was just 14, Dad had woken up just after me and proceeded to instruct me to get prepared for him to take me up to the Anjou (our neighbourhood) Shopping Center to get a haircut. Fourteen year olds tend not to take too cooperatively to such demands by their parents. The Beatles were all the rage back then and popularity, personal image and appearance was ever important to the era's youth. Fourteen was an extremely sensitive age and I had decided a few months back that my hair was a crucial and integral part of me, my image, my personality and my desired appearance. In fact, while attending high school, my hair length also played a fundamental role in my popularity. In other words, I had a different view of what was going to happen to my hair that day.

I had always respected Dad's instructions and good advice and guidance on such issues as hygiene, tidiness and appearance but peer pressure and self image had overtaken good sense as far as hair length went in those days and more and more of the guys at school were growing their hair to varying lengths. My hair had grown to perhaps 16" overall and I particularly wanted it long at the back. I had started playing guitar and was envisioning the days of performing with our band and simply felt I wanted to look the part. Popularity in high school was paramount.

Well, Dad continued to persevere and was determined I was going to get a haircut that Saturday morning. As he pulled on his sweater and grabbed his wallet and car keys, I took off ahead of him, darted out the front door and ran up the street, heading towards the boulevard that took us down to the tennis courts behind the French elementary school. The courts were supervised by Fred, a terrific black French man, hired by the city to tend to the courts and put up the nets each morning and take them down and put them away at night.

Fred was a nice, personable man who kidded with us and encouraged us to play tennis and occasionally played a few sets with us. He and his oriental friend, Bill, particularly enjoyed playing tennis with my Mom and Dad. It was my Mom and Dad and Fred and Bill who taught and encouraged me and my friends to play tennis, which ended up being my main and favourite sport for many, many years after moving to Ottawa.

So, that day, I ran to the back of the school, said hi to Fred and ran inside the back doors of the school into the gymnasium where a little locked room atop the stage stored the school's basketballs and volleyballs. I climbed over the walls of the storeroom and hid quietly among the balls, anticipating that maybe Dad would soon appear at the courts, looking for me and to take me to get a haircut. I had explained to Fred in my then limited French what was going on with my Dad and he had agreed to keep our secret about my hiding place. Before long, Dad appeared at the rear of the school, looking for me. I heard him bellow: P-E-T-E-R! P-E-T-E-R! I was very excited and intent on not getting caught, nearly peeing myself, all the while maintaining my silence among the balls, avoiding detection. Dad and Fred exchanged a few pleasantries with Dad eventually realizing the futility of his search. Dad must've then gone home and I remained at the courts, eventually going home at around 4:30. I thought that this was a safe time to confront Dad, still determined that I was not going to get a haircut that day. Well, as I walked into the house, Mom must have been preparing supper, and Dad saw me and immediately ordered me to come with him and scoot up to the barber shop before it closed in the next 15 minutes.

Well, I'm sorry to say that a heated argument ensued between us and I continued to firmly state my position. I usually always had regarded my parents' instructions and wishes but I guess I had reached that magic age where I wanted and needed to express my own preference with regard to my personal appearance. After all, I was a teenager and it was the late '60s. Our difference of opinion got quite involved but we remained communicative and fortunately Dad eventually conceded and I never did get that haircut. In fact, that was the last haircut I was ever asked or told to get. I guess I had reached that age. The picture below will give you an idea of the hairstyle I ended up sporting over the ensuing seven years. This is a picture taken by the Renfrew Mercury during a Tennis Tournament in which I played in 1971. I didn't win, by the way!

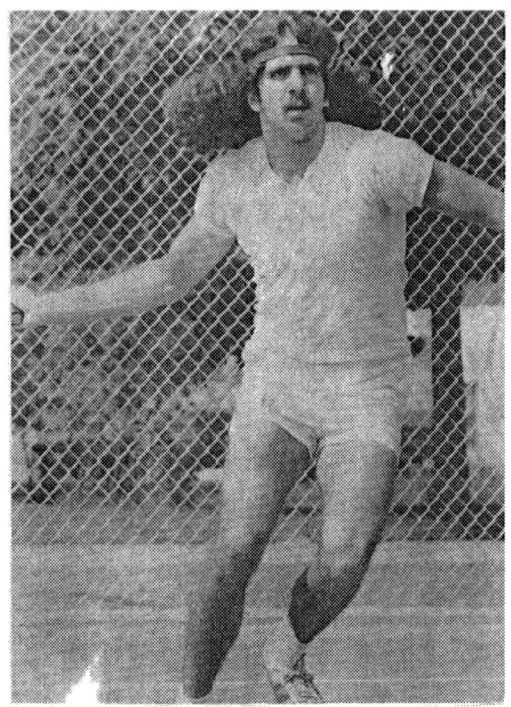

On the courts, Renfrew ca. 1971

CHAPTER 5:   MAN AND HIS WORLD

1967 was a magical year. Mom and Dad had bought me a season's pass to Man and His World (Expo '67), the World's Fair that was held in Montréal that year. I had turned 14 that March and was all set for the adventure of my life. The Mayor of the City of Montréal, Jean Drapeau, had successfully bid for, won and hosted a world class attraction that everyone enjoyed and appreciated.

In addition, Montréal had just completed construction of a number of arteries of its subway system, called Le Métro and it became quite easy and convenient to jump on a city bus, ride down to the Atwater Métro station and take a subway over to Ile Ste Hélène (St. Helen's Island), the hub of much of the attractions of the '67 World's Fair.

Expo '67 coincided with Canada's 100th anniversary of "Confederation". Its six month run drew 50 million visitors, mostly those under 40 years of age. It was an international exhibition that featured over 90 foreign, provincial, industrial and various "theme" pavilions.

The setting was beautiful, off of and surrounded by the St. Lawrence River, with many pavilions and exhibits at Ile Notre-Dame, the main island. Ile Ste Hélène represented a kid's dream as this was the location of the fair's amusement park, La Ronde. There were many rides and attractions. One of the significant rides I recall was the Gyrotron, a futuristically designed ride into a dragon's mouth way up high above the ground. Of course, there were also many international shops that we browsed through and where we sampled the various countries' chocolate, soda pop and cigarettes.

We rode thrill rides, shuttles and monorails all around the sites. There were two main islands and theme areas throughout the entire fair. I remember so clearly that year, the pavilions, the rides, the shops and the exhibits. It was like a magical dream world, a great place to visit as often as I wanted during its six month run for only $35.00, what a bargain! There was enough to see and do there 'eight days a week!'

CHAPTER 6:   MAGICAL PLAYGROUND

As I mentioned earlier, my friends and I frequently hung around the tennis courts behind the Ernest Crépault French elementary school in Ville d'Anjou. The school yard in the rear where the courts were installed was totally fenced and the woods bordered it to the south.

Before Mom and Dad eventually moved us to Ontario, we lived in Ville d' Anjou. From 1958 to 1971, we played for hours in the woods there, mostly riding our bikes around the endless bike paths that wove all around the bushes and trees, creating a magical, surreal and endless playground.

Later, as we approached and lived through our teens, we hung around the woods, sitting on fallen trees as we chatted and laughed with friends, drank pop or beer, smoked and bummed cigarettes. We often sat on the concrete steps of the west side of the school. The steps at the rear were the ones where the tennis court attendant, Fred, posted himself to monitor and control the installation and use of the tennis nets. Good ol' Fred put those nets up every morning and turned off the lights and took the nets down each evening just in case it rained. I tell you, there was a certain quality to life in those days and we sat on those rear steps with Fred for hours as he spoke his Caribbean French to us and we learned from him. I would say that hundreds of tennis balls ended up being hit over the rear fence, into the woods at the southernmost baseline of the courts. A good percentage of the balls also ended up on the roof of the gym at the eastern edge of the courts.

This roof had been atop a humungous wall which, I would venture to guess, was at least 40' tall where the gymnasium was. So, to get the errant tennis balls from up there, we had to first climb the lower section of the school via the drain pipes conveniently situated along the south wall, then we scurried up a metal ladder to get to the gymnasium rooftop. After a typical death-defying climb, we usually found at least 20 or 30 balls. The climb down from such a height was usually the most unnerving. We did this a few times each summer with, fortunately, no one ever getting hurt or plummeting to the ground.

CHAPTER 7: FIRES, FIRES AND BIGGER FIRES

When I was a kid, living in Ville d'Anjou in Montréal, we lit fires in the woods. Then, when I was a little older and approaching adolescence, we lit BIGGER fires in the woods. At the time, we were just kids needing something to do. We weren't juvenile delinquents or troublemakers and we never did any harm to anyone or anything. Also, we never stole or disrespected anything that wasn't ours and, in spite of our escapades, we never got arrested or had to spend any time in police custody. Okay, so we occasionally raided a few gardens and picked the Lorties' cherry and plumb trees.

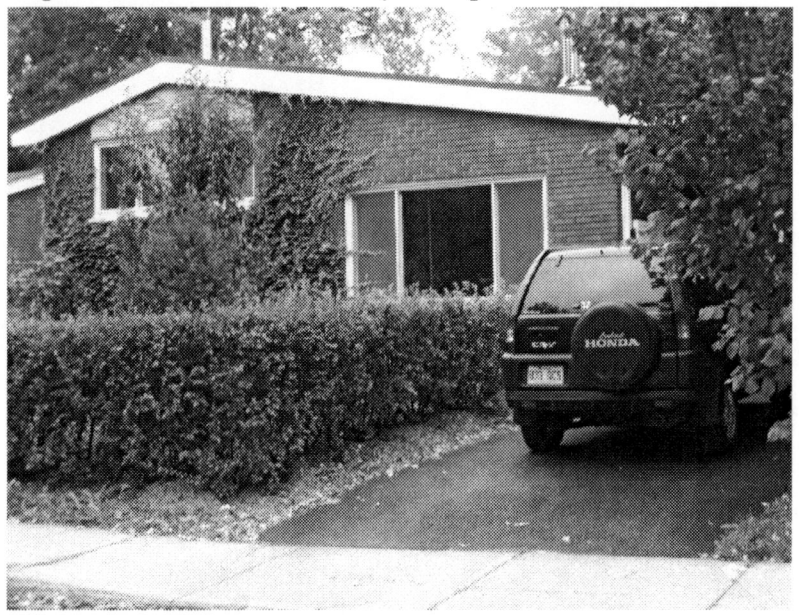

The house in which I grew up from 1958-1971 in Ville d'Anjou, Québec

I do recall that once or twice we received lectures from the police. We would be sitting on the curb of one of the neighbourhood streets, a police cruiser had pulled up to question us on our activities of the previous couple of hours and the police officers had eventually just driven away, satisfied that we were only just a few bored, harmless youths with nothing to do. I wasn't usually ever with my younger brother and sister during any of these episodes but I do suspect that some of their activities were similar to mine, as I learned over the years.

One morning and afternoon, my friends and I had collected branches, leaves, twigs and sticks from the forest floor and had made the hugest pile of timber, cardboard and brush we could stack, if you could imagine. Then, as dusk approached, we lit the bonfire. It could be seen for miles and before long, you could hear the sirens of the fire trucks. The forest was simply an area of pre-housing development and was just a lightly wooded scattering of trees and brush, not terribly dense and had numerous bike paths and tree houses built by kids from the immediate area.

We spent hours playing in these woods, driving our bikes and hanging around in them for years, up to our latest teen years when we would drag in 'cases of 24' from the nearest dépanneur (French for convenience store) and drink beer until dusk when the mosquitoes would drive us inside either to someone's home or the nearest bar. A couple of us were fortunate enough to look old enough and pass for the legal age and could get into the liquor stores and beer stores and be served beer or even get into the odd tavern or bar.

If we ended up in any of a few favourite taverns or bars, we would play Tibbits for hours.

So I attended high school in Montréal with the greatest of friends but no steady girlfriends. I was sort of popular in school just hanging around with the guys, usually sitting on the wall of the Texaco service station at the Anjou Shopping Centre, just outside Perrette's, our favorite "dépanneur" where we bought our "smokes" and pop. I always had someone to hang out with and bum cigarettes from and then, on weekends, we would go for beers at Joe's Bar and Legault's Tavern on Sherbrooke Street in the east end of Montréal. It was usually a contest to see how much draft beer we could drink; pretty cheap at just 20¢ a glass plus 05¢ tip! If we saved up $3.00 of our lunch money during the week, then we could buy 12 glasses of beer and stagger home after the bus ride there. Also, I remember how, in 1967, we would go to "Man and His World" (or Expo '67, as it was affectionately called) on weekends, mostly because my parents had bought me a season's passport for a mere $35. What an experience! We would visit all the countries' pavilions and we could buy cigarettes from every country! The Russian ones were oval-shaped and tasted awful, similar to the American ones. The Bell Canada pavilion was our overall favorite, however.

CHAPTER 8: ROCK CONCERTS

When I was 15, 16 and 17, I was going to all the rock concerts. The first concert I ever went to was The Beatles on September 8, 1964. The concert was at the Montréal Forum and my ticket cost a mere $5.50. I was only 11 years old, so my Mom accompanied me. Over the next few years, I also saw Led Zeppelin, The Who, Jethro Tull, Black Sabbath, Santana and Grand Funk Railroad. I lived for music. I remember experiencing Led Zeppelin on a powerful high quality stereo cassette deck that my Dutch friend Peter's father had. It was so awesome! The sound was magical! There was no turning back. I was hooked! Music was in my life to stay!

As I have mentioned, I am writing about my life because I nearly died. Now, it seems as though I have another lease on life. As I sit here in my wheelchair this afternoon, writing on my bed next to my snoozing wife, I think about how awe-inspiring my life was and still can and will be (this is my determination and also must be yours). My wife helps me want to go on. She is so wonderful and is everything to me. She loves me so much! Even her Mom, her Dad and her step-mom love me, and of course I love them all so very much too. They speak to each other on the phone nearly every day, keeping in touch and updating each other with gossip and news. My mother-in-law still lives in Montréal near her friends and family. This allows me the occasional opportunity to drive into my old neighbourhood of Anjou. Plus, we can visit our good friends Mike and Marie, who also live in Montréal near my mother-in-law. (We affectionately call my mother-in-law Gangan.)

As I said, I should be dead, after the hemorrhagic bleeds I had when I had my strokes. My short-term memory is a little screwed up, but still works and Hélène and I keep noticing that my long-term memory works very well as this writing should prove. I guess my I.Q., perceptiveness and cognitive abilities are relatively unaffected by my brain damage because I continue to show strong evidence that I have good logic and reasoning and I do pretty good on the PC and can perform simple household jobs which was always a hobby of mine. I have all the basic tools and love to tinker and fix things. I was pretty good with wires and electrical stuff, I guess encouraged from the days when I worked in Cable TV and I learned basic electronic fundamentals. I am limited in my physical ability for the time being however, because my left hand doesn't work and I could injure myself if I'm not careful.

So, back to the days in Montréal… I had a few best friends that I always hung around with, mostly John, Derek, Phil, Brian and Kenny. We were very loyal to each other and we knew how to laugh and have a good time. I was exposed to a few tragedies during my teens. My good friend Herman, who was the drummer in my band at the time, although we were constantly breaking up, took his life one Sunday night. I got a phone call from one of the band members to say that Herman had put a shotgun to his head and ended it! Another friend, Calvin, was from Renfrew and, at the incredibly young age of only 17, he went through a similar thing, not too sure what to do about girls and his popularity. One Sunday night, he decided to shoot himself while at home with his parents. These events were so sad and such a life lesson. The miles and years between the two incidents were considerable though, but the details surrounding them were almost identical. They were both young, good looking guys who loved music and girls and had written many poems to reflect on their lives, youth and foolishness. They had both been seeing girls at the time of their deaths and were fairly popular. I guess at some point they just got confused and disappointed with themselves and withdrew from the solid friendships they had.

Both occasions were surreal experiences where my friends and I were exposed to the grim realities of life and death. I ended up being a pallbearer at both funerals. Some of my closest friends and I were extremely supportive to the parents and the families in both instances.

CHAPTER 9: NOTHING'S GOING TO CHANGE MY WORLD

In 1970, when I graduated from high school, my parents moved us to Renfrew, Ontario, where I began another absolutely amazing chapter of my life. Yes, this is now all important to me and my damaged brain. I apologize to those readers I have lost or if I am boring you. I am hoping this book is a little entertaining to some of you who were either involved in or can relate to any of this reflection.

Anyway, as I was saying, the summer I graduated from high school I got together with two of my best friends and we set out on a hitchhiking trip to the east coast with Newfoundland as our ultimate destination. We got a ride from my Dad to the edge of Montréal at the Louis-Hypolite Lafontaine tunnel and John, Derek and I began to take rides from anybody who would stop and pick up three relatively clean-cut 17 year old young men, our thumbs out as we ventured along the Trans-Canada highway.

Our first ride was from a business woman traveling alone who spoke only French and who happened to be pregnant. Only John could speak any decent French so conversation was limited. We made it as far as Québec City before she dropped us off. I accidentally created a bit of an incident during our ride. When Dad had dropped us off just before we were picked up by this driver, I had tossed a brown paper bag lunch my Mom had prepared for me into the trunk of the woman's car. As we were let off at the end of our ride, near a hotel where this woman was to make a presentation, I naturally grabbed what I thought was my lunch. Well, that was a fatal mistake!

John, Derek and I got out of the car, thanking the woman and admiring her courage for picking up three strangers at the side of the highway. We had placed our backpacks on the shoulder of the road and prepared to put our thumbs into action and attempt to hitch our next ride. As we organized ourselves, I peeked into my backpack where I had placed my lunch bag and proceeded to look into it to take out a mid-day snack. To my utter surprise and amazement, I immediately discovered that the bag was not my lunch but a bag of cables and a microphone that was obviously the woman's presentation equipment. Derek and John cursed at me for the blunder. Derek was particularly nervous and irritated at me for initiating a shaky start to our adventure. I took a magic marker out and scribbled an explanation and an apology on the bag and planned to give the bag to a possible passing QPP highway patrol car.

Conveniently, before we had a chance to put my plan in action, the woman who had picked us up appeared, having gotten to her hotel, opened her trunk, discovered the missing equipment and turned her car around to come back and see if she could find us. Well, I tell you, I was so embarrassed and I apologized profusely. I gave her back her equipment, she drove off, and we resumed our thumbing towards the east coast.

CHAPTER 10:   YOUTH HOSTELS

One of our stops along the way on our hitchhiking trip out East found us in Rivière-du-Loup, Québec. We stopped that day to register to stay the night in the local youth hostel, where we fed ourselves with the usual 'help-yourself' hamburger, lettuce, tomatoes and, of course, condiments. We bunked in a gymnasium furnished with dozens of bunk beds for as many as 50 or more people. There were actually two separate bunk rooms, separating the males and the females. You must imagine that there weren't too many regulations at these accommodations; rough-housing, noise and promiscuity were strictly discouraged; the maximum stay was usually limited to only two or three nights; lights were to be turned out with all quiet by 11:00 pm and guests were discouraged from wandering or roaming near or outside the building after that time. Check-out time was supposed to be 11:00 am and a breakfast of bacon, eggs, tomatoes, cheese, bread and all the milk we could drink was supplied and left for us to prepare for ourselves. We had to be gone for sure after we ate and no one could remain in the building for lunch. While we stayed in the hostel, it was usually quite easy to make some quick, temporary friends. Some would sometimes have a guitar and we could get together over a Joni Mitchell, Neil Young or Beatles tune. I remember I had purchased an Eric Clapton songbook in a music store at a previous night's stopover and we spent a couple of hours strumming away to Badge, White Room and a few other of the rock legend's famous tunes. We were up until at least 2:00 am, puffing away at cigarettes and guzzling the supplied Coca-Cola but soon restlessness, impatience and boredom made us decide to go for a stroll up the street, into town.

When young people are given the opportunity to get out and travel and go away on an adventure, you can never be sure exactly what antics are likely to occur. One can only hope that we would stay on the right side of the law and that no one would get hurt.

Well, fortunately, that's exactly how this adventure unfolded. No one was arrested and no one got hurt!

After walking the streets for about a mile, our small group of about six males found ourselves in a quaint residential neighbourhood. To the right was a property with a nice wood frame house and a seemingly untidy rear yard. The front of the property was a huge, steep hill with the house at the crest. We painstakingly climbed the hill, puffing as we reached level ground at the house, the yard cluttered with junk such as old washing machines and appliances, a few rusty old cars, a couple of tire rims and some huge tractor tires, maybe 48" in diameter or larger. Our eyes lit up as we noticed the tractor tires. A couple of us moved toward them and started to attempt to stand them up, all the time imagining how easily and quickly they would roll down the hill if we stood them up, aimed them and gave them a gentle push. As is typical of young males, we were excited to the point of chuckling and nearly peeing ourselves and we lined up and prepared two or three tires to stand them up and launch them down the hill. I need to mention here that it wasn't only the prospect of rolling these tires down this property owner's hill that intrigued us but also that, at the bottom of the hill, the roadway continued at a considerable decline for quite a distance. I guess we had unscientifically calculated that the tires would possibly continue to roll down the street for a couple of miles. Of course, we never even considered what obstacles could possibly interrupt the path of these projectiles.

So it took two of us to huff and heave and lift and stand up each tire and we carefully aimed them toward the roadway at the bottom of the hill. We watched the tires quickly pick up speed and immediately realized the potential extent of the mischievousness we were engaged in and started to run down the hill and up the street so as to avoid any possibility of being caught in our fun. The evening ended without consequence. Phew!

One of our subsequent overnight stops was in Fredericton where we stayed at a youth hostel and simply had the time of our lives. We had rendezvous'd with a number of young people who obviously just wanted to party. We had secured overnight accommodation in Fredericton, where we were billeted in the student dormitories at the University of New Brunswick. The accommodation had been closed to the students for the summer and was reserved exclusively for the anticipated masses of transients that the Canadian government had budgeted and prepared facilities for that year. The student dormitories were made available to the hitchhiking population and were truly a luxurious scale of accommodation for such a group. Every night was an adventure as cases of beer, bottles of apple cider and the odd nickel bag of home grown was secreted into the dormitory hallways. Then we continued to the southern extremity of New Brunswick at the Bay of Fundy.

Within the first week, the three of us split up because we were bickering too much and driving each other crazy and we continued our adventure separately, with new people that we met along the way. I had the most incredible journey that summer that a young person could possibly experience at that age. It was safe to hitchhike in those days and we met many new people and did many crazy things throughout our trip. Mostly we stayed in youth hostels that usually cost under $1.00 a day and included a clean bed, bacon, eggs and milk for breakfast and usually unlimited hamburger and fixings for dinner. They didn't expect you to be there for lunch because the whole concept was that you were usually a transient just needing a place to crash for the night! I finally ended up back in Montréal, and I then took a Voyageur bus over to Ottawa, where I met my Dad and joined the family at our new home in Renfrew and continued my life in Ontario.

CHAPTER 11: A WONDERFUL NEW LIFE

Moving to Renfrew was the beginning of a wonderful new life. My Dad, Mom, brother and sister and I had just moved to this thriving metropolis (kidding) from Montréal where we had lived in a neat east end community for 13 years. Talk about culture shock! We had moved from this huge city of over 2 million to a rural town of only 8,500 and had to quickly adapt to the routines of new schools and new friends. I must say that the whole process was an absolute pleasure. Gerard, my first friend in town, had come over to introduce himself while I was working on our roof. We chatted and shared histories for a bit and before we were done, he had invited me to a party that evening, something that he did very well and often. With good ol' Gerard, there was always a party and he was the one who always had the most complete information of where and when it was happening that night and who was going to be there.

You see, Gerard was the best dressed young man in town. He worked for Frasier's, a men's fine clothing store, and would always be the one to see up the main street for the latest information on the parties happening that night. I had been exposed to the town for 24 hours and I can honestly say that I never had a dull or quiet evening for the next year. 1971 was a great year and, at 18 years of age, Renfrew was a good place to be for my Coming of Age! In this writing, I am finding that, due to my brain injury and associated memory deficit, I am actually reliving this time in incredible detail and having a ball doing it! Every night, any combination of Gerard,

Donnie, Garry, Terry, Gerry, Norm, Chris and myself would get together, finish a few cases of beer or a couple of bottles of Alcool and then head off to Butson's "Pits", suitably primed and ready for an evening of laughs and frolic.

One of the uncanny things I remember and cherish the most is how well I got along with all my friends' parents. I guess I was a good kid but could've been a bit of an uncertain thing when observed from afar. As you can see from my tennis picture on a previous page, I wasn't exactly the most well groomed lad in town. At that time, I was just off the boat from Montréal, so to speak, a fact that some of the folks in town didn't exactly know how to take. I didn't do drugs, but I enjoyed beer; I didn't smoke and, like John, Gerard and some of my other friends, I was pretty personable. Some of my friends' parents actually welcomed me and accepted me as a good example to their sons. I was proud of this and always enjoyed visiting and socializing with them. What was refreshing is that my Renfrew friends were all from good families and were honest and stayed out of trouble.

Also, most Friday nights, we would have the weekend warm-up at my house or sometimes at another friend's house. This usually involved six to ten of us cracking open a 40 oz. bottle of Alcool and mixing it with Tang orange crystals. After killing the 40 pounder, we headed off to the men's room at Butsons' where we enjoyed playing shuffle board, a few games of pool and some darts and, of course, drank "a few" cheap draft beer. Usually we were Gerard, Garry, Gerry, Norm, Donnie, Terry, Chris and a few others who were, off and on, a regular part of the gang. We occasionally played Tibbits, a cool game I had learned in my tavern days back in

Montréal and had introduced to the Renfrew lads. The game was played with two against two. You would tap and push a quarter from one end of the table to the other, trying to get as close to the edge as possible without going over and carefully hanging off the edge of the table partway so that you could flip and catch it. We played for hours and left the tavern many drafts later.

Of course, there was the time a few of us drove to Ottawa and visited the Museum of Science and Technology. We thought we had gotten on the unfamiliar Highway 417 toward Montréal, but actually were on Highway 17 heading toward Rockland and saw the sign directing us past Orleans. Being the country bumpkins that we were, we actually thought we were headed toward New Orleans in the U.S.! That day, we ended up driving to the He & She Hair Salon, where I had made an appointment. It was an upscale salon in Ottawa at which men and women went out of their way to get their hair cut and styled. We got there rather late in the business day and it eventually became obvious I was going to be the last customer of the day. The stylist robed me up and began to snip at my considerably long locks. I needed this haircut and she knew it! We had a friendly appointment, chatting the whole time, then casually but out of the blue she said to me "Hey, man, I happen to have something here that a friend brought in to me earlier. Would you like to share this Hash Brownie with me?" Honestly, I was not sure what to expect or what I was up against, but it seemed harmless and innocent enough. She was a pretty young thing and we seemed to be getting along well, so I said "Sure, what the hell!" and we nibbled away at the moist, fresh, aromatic cake. Before long, we were done the cake and soon, she was finished my hair. Being the shy but charismatic person that I guess I was, the pretty stylist asked me what I was doing later. Her day was over, but I had to tell her that I was headed back to Renfrew and had a car load of friends that were waiting for me to finish this appointment so I could drive them back to town. We expressed our mutual disappointment, I paid my bill, we said "See you again, sometime" and so ended my fantasy. I did start to drive, then gave the wheel to Gerard because the brownies were turning out to be of particularly good quality and my experience that day was epitomized.

CHAPTER 12:   THE MOD SQUAD

Terry called on me one afternoon and told me that he had discovered a young transient who had been attempting to push drugs onto elementary school children, in front of their school. Terry had picked him up hitchhiking along the main street in Renfrew and they had started talking while driving up the street when, all of a sudden, the punk asked Terry to pull over while he had a chat with some kids in front of their elementary school. That did it for Terry. Later that afternoon, he drove up to my house, where we concocted the most incredible scheme. You see, Terry knew the Chief of Police personally, Renfrew being the small town of 8,500 that it was.

Terry called Police Chief Wark and explained the incident he had witnessed with the punk and the drugs. What Terry was motivated to do then was to set up a 'sting' operation, where Terry and I would actually loan this punk about $40 to help him buy some more dope and we would then drive him up the highway to a reknowned drug distribution house in Arnprior so he could make his purchase. The exciting part was that Police Chief Wark had agreed to have a squad of patrol cars intercept us along the highway from Arnprior, driving back to Renfrew so the dude could continue his revolting deed. The punk, of course, was totally oblivious to our plan and Terry and I drove homeward in the front seat of his family's station wagon, fully anticipating the police cars that would be pulling us over at any moment.

We were on our way home, our eyes flitting to the rear view mirrors to observe the early stages of the coordinated interception. Our passenger seemed to be nervously craning for a better look at the peculiar official activity that was materializing behind us. Suddenly, his paranoia overcame him and he indicated to us that we were being followed. We attempted to downplay the obviously developing activity and our nervous passenger finally opened a window. We noticed the cruiser's emergency lights illuminating our rear view and we heard a brief burst of siren indicating for us to pull over as our passenger prepared a bag of something in his lap. Moments later, as our entourage sped up to direct us to the side of the highway, our buddy tossed something out the window. As an officer appeared beside our car, his eyes nervously yet knowingly looking right into Terry's and my eyes, I darted my gaze toward the rear of the car, trying to secretly signal to the officer that something had been tossed out behind the car. To be perfectly honest, at this point we truly did not know exactly what sort of character this drug-pushing low-life was. Did he have a gun, or maybe a knife? Had we been watching too much Mod Squad?

Anyway, we promptly pulled the car over and the officers routed Terry and I to one squad car and cuffed and took the punk to another car. That was the last we ever saw of our transient so-called friend. The police who had taken Terry and I drove us to the Renfrew police station, had coffees waiting for us in the interview room, shook our hands and thanked us. We chuckled and said goodnight, knowing the pusher was locked up, in the process of being charged. Talk about an exciting and satisfying night! We never did get our $40 back. We just considered it money well spent.

CHAPTER 13:   CLOSE CALL

It was a typical Friday night in Renfrew in 1971 and a number of the buddies and I had been talking about heading over to the Québec side to party at the popular Riverside Hotel over there. Or maybe we'd even go over to Bryson, a more happening place, with a little more rock'n roll and a little less country music. It was a particularly special day, however. Dad had brought home a used good condition Plymouth Fury to be my Mom's car and our official second family car actually for her and me to share. Dad had parked it in the driveway for Mom and me to excitedly admire and Mom took it for the first drive and blessed it with her seal of approval. We were more than happy. The car was special to her because it was her vehicle to get her up to the golf course one to four times a week to play golf with her girlfriends. It was special to me as I had just obtained my driver's license at my birthday the previous March and the car was to be available to me occasionally and as often as I could put gas into it. That Saturday morning, I took the car out and purchased an eight-track cassette player at the local Canadian Tire and spent the rest of the day installing it. There is something special and magical about the smell of new electronics being installed in a new car, even if it was second-hand. To Mom and me, it was new and grand!

That Saturday night, I asked Dad if it would be okay to take the car out to drive my friends and me to the hotel, which was up the River Road from Renfrew. We listened to some Supertramp and Chicago tapes at full blast on the ride over the Ottawa River to the hotel. I was in heaven with my new wheels. It took about 35 minutes to get to our destination, safe and sound. The trip back that night was similar but with one significant difference. We took the same route back but had a little incident along the way. While driving westbound along the River Road, we came to a sharp curve in the road which was signed to reduce speed to 30 mph. This was during the days of "miles per hour" rather than "kilometers per hour", so it meant to reduce for the turn from 50 to 30 mph or to 50 kilometers from 80 kilometers per hour. As I entered the curve, I was still doing the main highway speed of 50 mph or 80 kph. Considering my relative driving inexperience, it turned out that I simply was going too fast as I executed the curve.

The next thing we knew, I had crossed the road and found myself driving into the opposite lane, on the left shoulder. I yanked the steering wheel sharply to the right to try to correct the turn. Although the next event happened too quickly and I didn't really remember how it happened, it seems that the car then struck a sign post, rolled over to the right, up and on to the right front roof pillar, crushing the roof and popping out the windshield, smashing and launching it over the front of the car, landing at the rear, avoiding traveling through the car and missing decapitating any of the five of us. The car then apparently rolled one complete overturn, landing squarely back on all four wheels. At the end of the roll and upon inspection, the front left tire was flat which was of significance when I was explaining the chain of events in court and defending the entire sequence. I simply concluded and blamed the whole incident on a blown-out tire. In reality, I think I was probably just driving too fast.

It was incredible that no one was injured and one of us, Danny, actually slept through the entire event, waking in absolute awe half an hour later. So the good news was that Garry, Gerard, Danny, Owen and I all survived and were totally unhurt.

The following episode was a little humorous. Danny, Garry and Owen caught rides into town from some friends who were driving by but had stopped to see if we were all right as they were about to pass us on their way home from the hotel. Gerard and I were waiting with the car, having told the others to please call the O. P. P. to file the appropriate report. I was not worried about the police coming as I hadn't been drinking and nobody was hurt. I may have been wondering what this was going to mean to my insurance but I suppose I was more worried about how disappointed my Dad and Mom would be. After all, it was the first time out really for my and my Mom's new car. I learned the next day that the car was actually a write-off. It wouldn't even start that night when I tried it. I discovered later that it actually would start if I slipped the automatic gear shift into neutral. The right fender and door were slightly crumpled and the roof was a bit crushed on the right front. Other than that, it was in pretty good shape or so I thought and tried to convince myself. Gerard and I waited for perhaps three or four hours having a couple of cigarettes, lying back in the front seat of the car with our feet protruding through the missing windshield.

A few of our friends returning from the hotel came to screeching halts upon slowing and coming up to our wrecked auto and seeing our feet sticking out the windshield. As you can imagine, they were thinking the worst and were relieved when they discovered our smiling faces and observed our shoulders shrugging glumly when they asked us how everyone in the accident was. Gerard and I were quite calm but some of our friends nearly panicked as they ran up to us and found us to be alright.

After a few of our friends had stopped and proceeded homeward, once assuring themselves that we were okay, first a tow truck came to tow the car away, then a police car pulled up and the officer had us crawl inside and provide the details for his report. I remember meeting the officer to this day. His name was Constable Cavanaugh and he was pleasant enough but I was pretty disappointed when he handed me a ticket charging me with careless driving. I was pleased eventually, however, as Dad hired a lawyer for me who actually helped me beat the charge and kept my license devoid of any demerit points.

The consequence was that I had to come up with the $250 deductible and repay my Dad for the lawyer plus I had to do without the luxury of that second family car until my Dad bought a replacement for Mom and me a few weeks later. I learned a few lessons about driving carefully, protecting my insurance and avoiding driver's license charges and demerit points.

CHAPTER 14:   THE GUINEA PIG

Every once in a while, tragedies happen to us, to our friends and to our loved ones. Some of these incidents are regrettable and never should have happened. Well, on this one particular evening, an event took place that should never have happened and a few of us ended up sore and sorry that it did happen.

One Friday night, Mom and Dad had gone out and had left me home to care for the house. I invited a few friends over to have a few beers and to listen to some music. The evening proceeded harmlessly enough and I was sitting in my bedroom downstairs having a few beers with a few friends. All of a sudden, I heard a commotion out in the recroom just outside my bedroom. A few people were shouting excitedly and I rushed out to discover that one of the guests had somehow got hold of my brother's pellet gun and shot my sister's pet guinea pig, which was in a cage in the far corner of the basement.

I flew out of the bedroom in a rage, seeing the culprit running up the stairs, heading for the front door. I suppose I was still just letting the grim reality of the incident sink in and I probably flew up the stairs two or three steps at a time, eventually catching up with the marksman and tackling him at the very top of the long stairway. The rest was a blur as I wrestled him to the ground, my fists flying, hopefully teaching him the lesson of his life. My sister was sobbing. She was the family vet-to-be and loved all animals so much. What was so disturbing about the incident was that someone had come into our home, albeit invited by me, and had had the nerve to disturb our peace and compromise our personal space and the sanctity of our family. I never saw the invader again after that but I was told that his injuries from the altercation were significant. That night, a number of us drove over to one of the local vets with the guinea pig, who was unconscious and bleeding from behind its ear. We walked up to and surrounded the vet's back door. Now, by the way, did I mention that all this was happening at about 1:00 am? The doctor was obviously in bed and I pounded on his back screen door with great determination, attempting to get him to pay attention to our urgent situation.

The vet eventually appeared at the door, opened it and admitted a couple of us to his downstairs treatment lab. He administered a shot of a painkiller or something humane and appropriate for such a situation. We soon walked up the stairs and outside, with me carrying the poor bleeding animal in a cardboard box, trying to think only of its possible recovery and how I could tell my sister that it was going to be okay. Well unfortunately, although we got the little pet back to the house, it was dead by the morning and grief and regret came over all of us. The next day was dismal and I apologized to my sister profusely. Fortunately, we eventually forget even the saddest of events and we move on.

CHAPTER 15:   LIFE GOES ON

Although I eventually got married to the most wonderful and most beautiful woman who coincidentally is also from Montréal, I actually met her several years later in Toronto and married her only just two and a half years ago. I get sad when I think of it but I wish I had known her back in the Montréal days and that we had experienced our teens and twenties together. We are such good friends and lovers now and would have been such wonderful friends then and we would have had so much fun together. Well, we are in our early 50's now and fortunately still are having lots of fun and enjoying our time together so much, despite my newfound disability. Anyway, you can't have your youth back; those years are long gone and are now history. But you can still enjoy your life.

After I finished grade 13 in Renfrew, Mom and Dad hustled me off to college in Ottawa. I enrolled in an Architecture program but eventually dropped out after learning a lot about the basics of house construction and design. That year, I ended up working for my Uncle Buzz, renovating cottages over on the Québec side in Norway Bay, coincidentally across the Ottawa River from Renfrew. I must mention the episode when the foreman had asked me to dig a septic tank in the damp sand. I had placed the first of about six frames of 2"x6"s in the ground and the objective was to start digging between them and lower those six frames to build the septic tank. After digging for about three hours, I finally quit and went home, never to return to the job. That was my first and last experience at hard labor! Another life lesson learned! My good friend Donnie heard that night that I had quit and he offered my uncle to continue the job. You know, even now, about 34 years later, we were laughing the other day at how he finished that septic tank and how much he had hated it. During a recent visit to Arnprior, we had a little reunion with some friends from the Renfrew days who still are wonderful friends. By the way, we have promised that we will do this again later this summer but with a few more of us because some were not able to make it this time. Why would we want to end a good thing?

I find that the best part of living in Renfrew is that, even though I only lived there for one year, the friends I made during that year have become and still are my lifelong friends that I will always treasure.

CHAPTER 16:   MADOC POP FESTIVAL

It wasn't quite Woodstock, but it was the next best thing. It was a Canadian attempt at being famous in the world of rock and pop music.

In 1972, I had been attending Algonquin College in Ottawa and had come home for the summer. In the midst of the new world in which I was living since my Mom and Dad had moved our family to Renfrew a year before, I joined two friends, Gerard and Eric, and made plans to drive in my friend Eric's van to Madoc, Ontario. Madoc would be the location of a fairly large pop festival that we had all heard much about and which we were eagerly anticipating attending. I remember it as being a significantly decent attempt at comparing or competing with the likes of the Woodstock Music Festival in 1968.

Actually, just before heading to the festival, Gerard, Eric and I drove to Port Elgin and Southampton, Ontario, just off Lake Huron, to visit another good friend, Terry. We were taking a summer break, touring and enjoying the province. Actually, Terry had been my best friend for a while after I first settled in Renfrew, and I became attached to and fond of his family. So, Gerard, Eric and I selected a day and visited and drank with Terry and then soaked up the sun and checked out the gorgeous bikini-laden beaches of Port Elgin and Lake Huron. We had a ball and partied there for a couple of days. Then, we packed up again and ventured across Southern Ontario highways, southward until we got to Madoc and followed the signs directing concert-goers to one of the many entrances to the site.

Lines of people of all ages wound their way into the festival grounds and music blasted its welcoming ring from hugely stacked speaker columns throughout the site. People ambled along, in some cases aimlessly, between tents and refreshment/concession stands. Almost everyone carried and was swigging on a beer from their personal stock, most likely secretly smuggled in past security staff in their coolers. I clearly recall that we got into the grounds with a Coleman thermos jug of what we called Kick-a-Poo Joy Juice, a homemade concoction of vodka, Galliano and orange juice.

Having arrived at the site and rendezvous'd with a group of friends from our little town who had also ventured to the festival, we gradually set up our tents and lean-tos on the first day and built many campfires around the music-saturated site. We had such a good time during that event.

As we initially parked our van and started our first tailgate party, we enjoyed our first few beers under the blazing sun. It was going to be a 'toaster' of a day. We were unpacking our gear and I was tossing some of our rudiments and camp equipment out onto the grass. I tossed an axe in John's direction and he growled irritably at me as it bounced over his leg and precariously close to his manhood. I responded apologetically and assured him there was no need to worry as it wasn't intended to land that close to him. The others, including my good friend, Jane (who, coincidentally, is John's sister and who is now married to Doug, a dear friend who eventually became Hélène's and my Best Man), chuckled at the incident and we all returned to our beverages, sitting comfortably on the van's tail gate.

The guys were getting their bits of entertainment as the occasional bare-breasted female pranced or scooted across the grounds. The guys were sliding along giant mud slides making a wild scene and having a riot, naked as jay-birds. At one particular moment, while we were enjoying the Stampeders' "Sweet City Woman", a strung-out sort of lad popped out of his tee-pee with conceivably the largest cigar-sized joint of pot we had ever imagined. He graciously passed it around to anyone and everyone who would take some. He was quite the hit. I was privately strumming "House of the Rising Sun" on my acoustic guitar for a small circle of 60s music fans.

The next few days were hot and long and each one eventually stretched into the dark of evening while the parties and revelry continued noisily until everyone faded into the night. On the last morning, we packed our gear and prepared for the trek outside the grounds and headed back to the 'Frew. As we drove homeward, Gerard, Eric and I reflected on our unbelievable past 72 hours' experience. We had a hard time actually believing all the adventures we had just been part of. We laughed in awe most of the trip back home and Gerard moaned in pain as he had the worse sunburn after a couple of wonderful days in the blazing sun.

It was just too bad that the scale and magnitude of this concert hadn't rated documentation and filming like Woodstock had. But I was able to look some of the joys of it up on the internet the other day, 33 years after it happened and I am now documenting and reliving some of it here, in these paragraphs of my book.

SECTION TWO – MOVING ON

CHAPTER 1: SPORTS, GAMES AND MORE GAMES

I was 42 and played tennis competitively in house leagues with my friends. I had moved to Ottawa in 1971 and started playing tennis in the local racquet clubs and became pretty competitive. I made a lot of tennis friends and started playing in the house leagues, doing pretty good, and winning my share of matches. There were lots of men to play with and I entered the tournaments and occasionally won them. Unfortunately, or fortunately depending on one's perspective, there were plenty of good players, so it was always a challenge to win. I guess I wouldn't have had it any other way, because it all contributed to how well I played. We had quite a group of good friends who all played rather well.

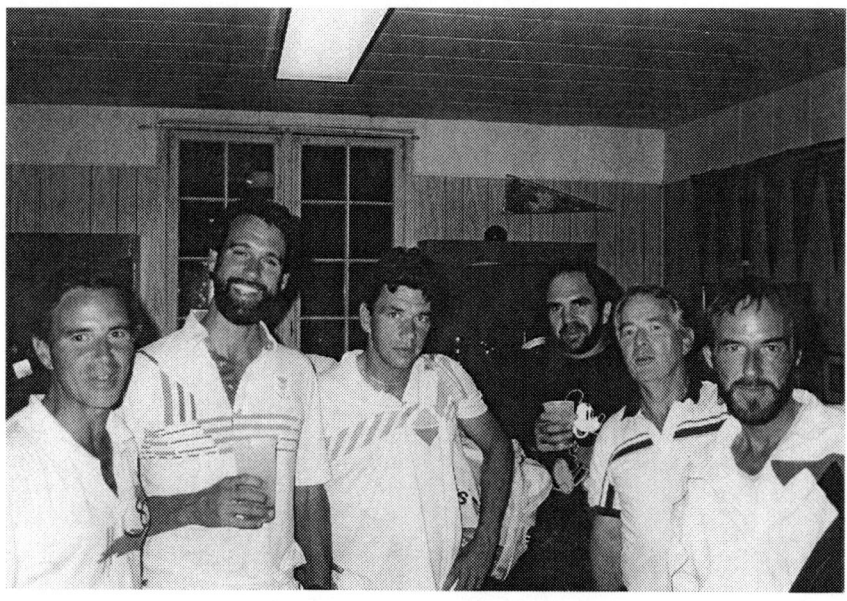

Ottawa Tennis gang, ca. 1980

The two tennis clubs that I frequented the most and at which I had memberships for many years, were the Ottawa Athletic Club ("The OAC"), mostly during the winter season and the Ottawa Tennis and Lawn Bowling Club – ("The Ottawa"), at which I played during the summer season only. It seemed that most of the guys that I played against were members of both clubs, so the competitiveness was a year-round thing for us.

Oh yes, about "The Ottawa". It was (and still is) an amazing club. At that time, it was managed by Gord and his brother Steph and during the last year I was there, before being transferred to Cornwall, Steve and I won the club "Intermediate", an annual tournament, which was always a challenging and "fun" event that created much rivalry and led to us consuming considerable pitchers of draft beer. To this day, I miss the camaraderie and the competitiveness and of course seeing and playing with my friends who were such good sports and good friends. I still have the trophies I won at these clubs, which are testimonial to some of the great fun and successful times I had on the courts. Cheers to you Jean, for the many tournaments we attempted, occasionally successfully and frequently frustratingly.

"Competitiveness", by the way, according to Dave, is spelled and pronounced "competiveness"! We all laughed over that one many times.

CHAPTER 2: NEWFOUNDLANDERS, PITCHERS AND GOOD COMPETITION

Between 1973 and 1979, I became intimately involved with the game of Fastball. Before I started playing tennis as proficiently as I did, during the first couple of years at my new cable job, I somehow got myself roped into coordinating the company fastball team. I was 20 years old when I started to play and we had organized and joined an industrial league team sponsored by my employer, Skyline Cablevision that first got me interested in playing Fastball competitively. This team started as an industrial house league team, and eventually developed into an intermediate "B" team as the league became more competitive albeit with my and Chuck's encouragement and guidance. Because I was so keen to play, I rallied some employees at work to become involved and become part of the sponsorship that Vic, our General Manager, had generously provided to help us organize, equip and uniform a team of about 12 of us. Some of us were enjoying playing and most were committed to participating and showing up for many of the games. Unfortunately, some of the players did not treat the schedule with too much respect. Quite often, only half of the employees would go out of their way and always show up only to discover that the other half were not taking the commitment too seriously and did not show up regularly. This forced us to forfeit many games and risk suspension from the league. This laziness was always a disappointment to all the other reliable and committed players, resulting in a considerable waste of time and embarrassment for those of us who wanted to play because such poor sportsmanship is usually not tolerated for long. So, those of us who had decided we wanted to take the game and the league a little more seriously decided that, in future, we would apply stricter governing house rules to the team. Réjean and I, as team managers, decided that all players would be expected to show up regularly and attend practices if they wanted to play. To miss a game or practice would result in players sitting out subsequent games. As time went on and in order to be reasonably competitive, we allowed players from outside our work unit to join the team and help us win games.

Fortunately, as players were told that they were to sit out for missing games or not showing up for practices, they began to be pissed off at what they thought were too strict and tight-ass rules so the non-committed ones eventually quit and we began to win more games, an overall more successful team. The players who never missed were more satisfied at the improved sportsmanship and felt the rules were fair and reasonable. Also, key to the amazing success we had with our 'ball' team were the Newfoundlanders and some Frenchmen we had at the core of the team. They were the best! At this time, if you wanted to build a good team, you were best off stacking it with Newfies. Of course, I always clearly remembered the time that Ronnie lined himself up one day at Kent's place and ploughed head first repeatedly into his metal garden shed, head-butting it possibly as many as ten or so times, denting it so that it was just never quite the same. Ronnie never scratched or harmed himself which was more than I could say for poor Kent's shed.

Also, I guess because I was enjoying playing so much and because I had learned to play fairly well, albeit at a relatively late age for taking up a competitive sport, I ended up becoming the league representative with the department of recreation for the City of Vanier, the municipality in Ottawa that provided and allocated our ball parks. I must say that our park, which was located right beside the Ottawa River, was the most gorgeous park site that you could imagine. There were two diamonds, covered in light sand, which were located beside the Rideau River and across the river from a row of gorgeous condominiums. As I became more involved with running the league and representing our group within the department of recreation, I organized and ran tournaments for a few years to help raise funds so that we could purchase and install a lighting system for the second of two diamonds and also to purchase and install fences for both diamonds and simply create a more complete ball facility. Before long, I became the league president and also helped run and coach the team with my good friend, Chuck. Chuck and I were the primary organizers for our league, working in cooperation with another men's Fastball league to hold a tournament each year and hopefully raise these funds. Collectively, we were successful in raising enough funds to go toward the lighting and fencing systems for the two diamonds. Chuck and I had a lot of fun and we worked hard to prepare and organize these tournaments. It was quite a feat to assemble as many as 32 teams for each tournament and collect sponsorship money and obtain beer sponsors. I suppose it was my organizational skills and Chuck's diplomatic ability that guaranteed that our events were successful. We partnered with many of our league's and our team's players such as Bob and John (the 'Hawk') to put together first class events. I can never forget the energy and man hours that went into these tournaments. And Chuck and Deb, I salute you guys. I love you.

Our team had some great players. We won many games and championships, thanks to the likes of pitchers Dwight and John.

I eventually quit as president of the league and quickly replaced this huge time commitment of fastball and its management and administration with tennis which I played four or five times a week for years thereafter. We had a great group of tennis friends who played together all the time at the Ottawa Athletic Club and the Ottawa Tennis and Lawn Bowling Club and before too long, we were all also playing golf, driving up to Hughie's chalet in the Laurentians each spring with Dave, Nigel, Owen and Bernie for our annual golf tournament. Mike conceived the "running drive" and Dave had the wickedest slice you could possibly imagine! You'll have to ask Bernie about the black flies and my legs! I can't emphasize enough how amazing these tennis clubs were and how much fun we had over the years. Ask Jean, Owen, Denis, Janet, Steve, Hughie, Bernie, Fred and others about how we would close the Ottawa Tennis and Lawn Bowling Club pub most nights.

CHAPTER 3: ONWARD AND UPWARD

I continued to take University courses after I started working in the Cable TV industry in Ottawa in 1973. I never graduated but I guess I had achieved a reasonable range of Business and Marketing credits which allowed me to make the progress I did over subsequent years in the different jobs and businesses with which I became involved.

In 1972, I was attending Algonquin College in Ottawa, having just completed grade 13 in Renfrew, after graduating high school in Montreal in 1970. That summer, after I had completed high school, I took off out east on a hitchhiking trip with two of my good friends, John and Derek.

In 1971, I found myself living in Ottawa, sharing a really cool townhouse downtown with some other friends who were at a similar stage in their lives: going to school, taking courses, having a great time and embarking onto the earlier stages of their respective careers. I never finished my program at college and decided instead to find a job and save some money to buy a car. I got a job at Cargo Canada on Merivale Road at Baseline Road. It was a poor-paying but fun retail clerk job. One day, a friend of mine, Ezzie, referred me to a man called Alfred Dodge. He was a large man, looking like a heart attack waiting for a time and place to happen. To this day, I am not sure what happened to him. It is so many years ago now. He was an interesting and nice man who at that time owned a small courier business. He offered me a really cool job running deliveries to many interesting locations in Ottawa, including the Federal Departments of External Affairs, Public Works and numerous other commercial locations such as A.B. Dick and Warners Ltd. It truly was a good and fair job because I was still just a young guy, mostly just looking to enjoy life and earn enough money to pay the rent, make the car payments and buy my groceries. I enjoyed the many parcel deliveries I made, going in through the back doors of so many business and government locations and talking to the cute girls with whom I would have to interface at each delivery.

But, as usual, all good things must come to an end. Actually, this time, there was a very good reason. My pay checks were bouncing! So, I decided to get out of that situation, lickety-split! I then decided to get serious about life and find a half-decent job. I decided that I was going to check with Bell Canada and the two cable companies in town and see if I could get hired as a technician or even try line work. Well, one afternoon, I was driving north on Saint-Laurent Boulevard in the east end of Ottawa and I looked over to the left and noticed the cable company office that serviced the east side of Ottawa. The company was called Skyline Cablevision and I drove into the parking lot, pulled up to the front door, went in and asked a girl there if there was somebody I could talk to about a job. She disappeared into some offices in the building and eventually came back and guided me to a technical office in the back of the building. The technical manager there, Tony, met me and we talked about the prospect of me working there. The job seemed exciting and I was certainly very interested. By the time our conversation was over, he had hired me.

CHAPTER 4:   LAKE PLACID 1980 WINTER OLYMPIC GAMES

I was a Maintenance and Quality Control Technician, working for an Ottawa area cable TV company, from 1973 to approximately 1991. In 1980, our General Manager bid on and won the contract for us to build and provide an in-house cable TV system for the venues at the 1980 Lake Placid Winter Olympic Games. What an exciting time that was for my colleagues and me!

Actually we were recruited as subcontractors for the local television network, CTV, who held the primary contract. We were fully responsible for building and installing the entire cable network which was designed by our Chief Engineer, Tony. The purpose of this system was to provide cable television feeds for the international commentators who would be providing the various nations' audio feeds to be simulcast with the host broadcaster ABC's main video feed.

Cable TV people are a breed apart. They are very hard working, competent and personable individuals and are very proud of their trade and workmanship. They are also quite renowned for knowing how to have a good time. Ask Larry, Bob, Denis and Terry, who had the job of installing the cables for the television monitors in the commentator's booths.

Our GM, Vic, was an excellent manager and a very personable and supportive man. He respected and treated his employees very well. Now, for this particular assignment, he had selected a number of us to work on this project, which we were all very excited about and pleased to be involved with. We were assigned in teams to work in Lake Placid one week at a time, of course with all expenses paid which included occasionally going to the finest hotels and restaurants in this exclusive tourist area. The whole experience was such an amazing opportunity because we were on the site of an international, high security, high profile event and had been granted absolute top security clearance and privileges where the countries' top athletes were gathering, practicing and preparing to compete.

Our clearances not only granted us access to good seats to the world's various hockey games but our passes even actually allowed us to lean right up against the boards of the hockey rinks and watch the games from the closest possible vantage point. We were at arm's length from all the action! Also, we were able to stand on the bridges that passed over the Luge and Bobsled tracks and get a bird's-eye view of those venues. Jean-Guy and I would go out each morning and inspect our job sites to make sure that the cable TV electronic equipment was working properly after sitting quietly unattended overnight. Talk about a sweet job. We were responsible for ensuring the systems we had installed were working each day. Never once did we find anything malfunctioning. We were paid to work the sites, nothing ever went wrong and the bonus was that we got to attend the Olympic events at no cost. We were satisfied and gratified at such an interesting and successful project.

We got to take some wonderful photographs. Be sure to look at some of my wonderful shots of Charlie, Jean-Guy and I working at the Olympic sites. Especially, do not miss the one of "THANK-YOU CANADA, FUCK YOU RUSSIA". What a historic moment that was!

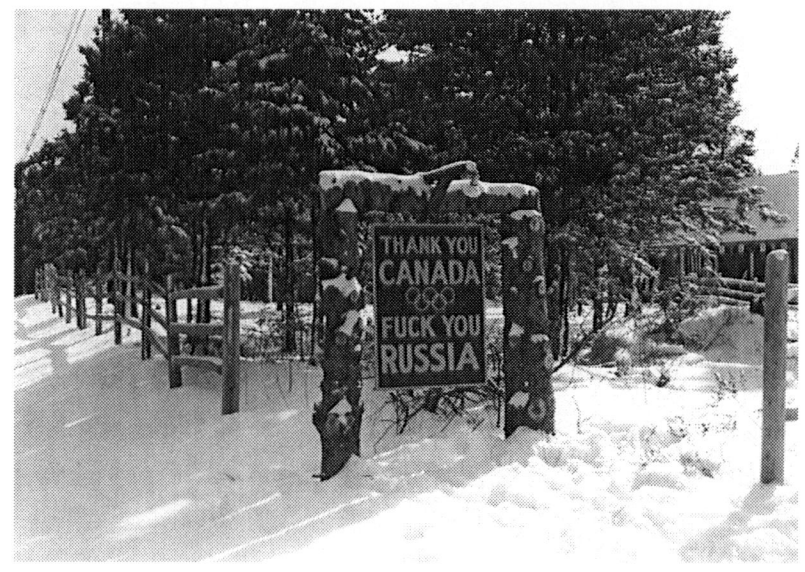

Winter Olympics, 1980 – Lake Placid, N.Y. (a historic moment)

Sixty-six Americans had been taken captive by Iranian student militants who had seized the U.S. Embassy in Tehran on November 4, 1979 to protest Washington's refusal to hand over the U.S.-backed Shah of Iran for trial. The original group included three diplomats who were at the Iranian Foreign Ministry. Six more Americans escaped. Of the 66 who were taken hostage, 13 were released on November 19 and 20, 1979; one was released on July 11, 1980, and the remaining 52 were released on January 20, 1981.

Six American diplomats avoided capture when the embassy was seized. For three months they were sheltered at the Canadian and Swedish embassies in Tehran. On January 28, 1980, they fled Iran using forged Canadian passports and an elaborate CIA scheme that had them posing as part of a film production company scouting for locations. The escape plan had been engineered by Ken Taylor, who was then Canadian Ambassador to Iran.

Eight U.S. servicemen from the all-volunteer Joint Special Operations Group were killed in the Great Salt Desert near Tabas, Iran, on April 25, 1980, in an aborted attempt to rescue the American hostages.

The reviled Shah of Iran, forced to flee Iran after the Islamic Revolution, had been admitted to a New York hospital for treatment and angry demonstrations against the United States had been held all weekend in front of the embassy.

For 444 days, the American hostages were held captive by radical followers of the Ayatollah Khomeini, fuelled by a hatred for America and a burning desire to re-establish Islamic ascendancy. Some of the hostages were hung by their wrists and beaten; others were subjected to terrifying mock executions.

But all made it home alive.

For Canadians, it was one of our finest hours. For the Americans, it was one of the darkest as the most powerful nation on earth was left impotent in the face of a new, unpredictable threat. And for the world, it was the beginning of the future.

The 1980 Lake Placid Winter Olympic Games proceeded peacefully from February 13 to February 24.

While driving to an inspection of the commentators' booths at the giant ski-jump site, Intervale, one morning, Jean Guy and I came across an official-looking sign with a rather rude and suggestive political message that had been erected overnight. We even attempted to drive past the sign again a little later and catch another look and take a few more pictures but we discovered it had been taken down, I guess by the local state troopers, before it created an issue with sensitive and important international visitors.

At this time in my life, as a Quality Control Technician for my company on this jobsite, my specific assigned duty on this project was to inspect and make sure the involved electronic components were always working properly each day, which they always were. Fortunately, with our frequent spare moments, we were able to go to the VIP hospitality areas and make sure the particular venue's TV and cable systems were in place and operational. Occasionally, we would have to go to the central equipment supply warehouse and stealthily acquire an available television set for one of the hospitality sites that happened to be in need due to some disorganization. We subsequently earned many Brownie points for our helpfulness and assistance and were usually pampered with a particular country's hospitality, including generous servings of hors d'oeuvres and refreshments. Gosh, actually, we were treated like VIPs! The hostesses were always pleasant and friendly and usually good-looking too.

CHAPTER 5: CORPORATE UPHEAVAL

I worked for Skyline Cablevision, an Ottawa area cable company, for 18 years, until they were bought out by Canada's largest cable company. It was then that my professional life took a drastic turn. Tragically, one day, the new owners came on site and fired all the senior management except for Tony and me. Much to my complete and utter surprise, one day a couple of my new superiors appeared at my office and announced to me that my former bosses and some other superiors were no longer with the company and that I was now to be the Division Manager or the senior head-honcho of the operation for which I had been working for the past 18 years. While I was very fortunate to have survived that corporate upheaval, it was truly a sad day, considering that many of my former colleagues were no longer with the company. To this day, I must say that I appreciated working with these people and am grateful to them for the wonderful years we had together.

Then, a few years later, I met an inevitable, similar fate as my former Skyline colleagues. I had five excellent years at the company that took us over, having been transferred initially from Ottawa to Cornwall as its Division Manager and then to Toronto as Manager of its Telemarketing operation. Fate soon caught up with me, however, when the company hired a new Call Centre manager who initially had a new telemarketing centre built, then fired me because I didn't fit his culture vision. How ironic that was because this manager also soon left the employ of the company. It seemed that he had just been hired to do their dirty work (fire me).

A few months later, after initially enjoying a good part of an attractive severance package, I ended up getting a terrific job with an exciting and successful music and video mail order business in the east end of Toronto. Once more, I worked with the most amazing and progressive senior management team. We communicated and worked together so well. In addition, I had the privilege of working with the most excellent U.S. head office team, including those responsible for the IT component of the organization with whom I liaised to coordinate the telecom and IT requirements for the Canadian side of the company. That was so enjoyable and rewarding because the individuals were so interesting and committed and such a pleasure to work with that they literally made the company the delight it was to work for. I especially want to acknowledge my good and special Indiana IT buddies, Dave, Rich, Don and Bob, not to mention the amazing Vaughan, my Canadian IT partner. Again, what an unfortunate shame it was that a good thing such as this company wasn't destined to remain the wonderful source of employment it had been. I extend many thanks and my unending gratitude to my former colleagues. Good luck guys!

Then, several years later, some unsettling news on the future of the company for which I was working began to circulate and it appeared to us as though it might be wise to consider alternate, more secure employment. A large corporate takeover seemed inevitable and the members of the senior management team were becoming a little nervous about their job security. Apparently my particular position as Senior Director of Customer Service, including managing the company's IT department, initially wasn't necessarily at too much risk. However, I had already been contacted by a head hunter on another exciting and attractive opportunity which I decided to consider and eventually accepted which, conveniently, turned out to be only ten minutes from my home.

It was really quite sad and unfortunate to part company with these wonderful people but the new company made me a decent offer and I decided to work with them. There, again, I worked with some very dynamic people for just a little over a year before I had my stroke. The president, Vaughn and vice-president, Bruce, were the most amazing executives, taking extremely good care of their people and conducting the most amazing motivational meetings and taking us out on the most incredible team-building sessions. One such event brought us to a Crosby, Stills, Nash and Young concert at the Skydome and another time, they brought us and our wives to a wine-tasting excursion at Niagara-on-the-Lake. The next thing we knew, the company was acquired by another large company, once more indicating uncertainty for an as yet to be determined few. I hadn't yet become part of any sort of planned corporate upheaval but I then became sick with a stroke before hearing of any such instability and was declared by my family physician as no longer fit for work. Thank goodness for Long Term Disability insurance!

During my working life, I was always professional, hard working and honest. I believe I was always a good example to my subordinates and was used to getting much positive feedback from both my peers and my superiors. I worked for some very dynamic and effective people. Some of them had been very fair superiors and I can truly say that I always looked forward to going to work. I enjoyed many business lunches and dinners throughout my professional life, always appropriately expensed to the company as legitimate work-related meals or entertainment.

I am also proud to say that I had some excellent and very capable supervisors and managers whom I worked with and for and who reported to me. I had a very positive and encouraging work ethic that I advocated to all my direct reports and, although it is approaching 30 years since I worked with some of them, I still hear from many of them today, usually by email, some of them still passing on some very flattering and complimentary comments about some of our experiences together years ago. Some of these very competent individuals that I was proud to have worked with include Denis, John, Harry, Kevin and Larry, going back to my Cable TV days as early as 1973 and working with Joan, Martina, Sylvie, Vaughn, Harjinder, Don, Rich, Dave, Ben and Elmo during my music company term.

My best friends and tennis and golf buddies, Dave, Owen, Nigel, Denis, Fred, Steve, Hughie, Mike and Bernie and I would spend countless hours arguing, laughing, drinking draft beer and encouraging each other on our respective jobs and careers which, I believe, drove us to our respective successes in the years that came and went.

During my terms with the companies for which I worked from 1973 to 1997, I became a volunteer associate on the Call Centre Council with the Canadian Marketing Association, which gave me the opportunity to work with some fascinating professionals and dynamic call centre entrepreneurs. This incredible experience allowed me to rub elbows at a board table once a month with the gurus who established the rules and guidelines for ethical and professional marketing in Ontario. Thank you, John, Bonnie and all.

Now, I am in a wheelchair with an indefinite recovery prognosis. I am living a nice, quiet life with my wife and son and our wonderful Golden Retriever, Cooper.

SECTION THREE – NO REPLY

CHAPTER 1:   I'VE JUST SEEN A FACE

Hélène and I met in January of 1997. We were introduced by a mutual friend who knew us both very well and who also knew instinctively that we had much in common and would probably hit it off.

Our first "date" wasn't really a date at all. Our friend, Robin, arranged for all three of us to go to a local karaoke bar to listen to some music and share a few laughs. I wasn't really looking for someone new in my life just then and neither was Hélène; in fact, we discovered some time later that we had both entertained thoughts of backing out of that evening. Imagine! Had we listened to the little voices inside our heads, we never would have met our respective soul mates. Thank goodness, for whatever reason, we connected and have been together ever since.

I was very shy as a boy growing up and, as a result, I was somewhat leery about meeting new people. Hélène was and continues to be a real "people person" and I found her easy to talk to right from the start.

When we met, Hélène had a 16 year old son, Paul and I had two boys, ages 11 and 6, named Tyler and Corey respectively. Coincidentally, we were both originally from Montréal, having moved to Ontario in the 70's. We liked the same music, the same sports and even the same types of social and athletic activities. All in all, a match made in heaven!

Before we knew it, the five of us were one big, happy family with Hélène and Paul moving into the home that my two boys and I lived in prior to our meeting.

Shortly after we met, my family physician began to monitor my blood pressure. He prescribed blood pressure medication (actually a fairly low dose initially) and I saw him regularly to monitor how effective the medication was. My life at the time was busy and active. I was living in the suburbs north of Toronto. I played in a tennis league at our local country club, dabbled in classic rock music and enjoyed a busy and rewarding social life. Hélène and I were both members of the same country club. Having moved to the Toronto area a few years prior, I made a point of visiting my family in the Ottawa Valley on a regular basis. My sons were still quite young at the time and Hélène and I were kept on the go every night with the kids' activities including baseball and hockey games and practices, Jiu Jitsu, music lessons, appropriate errands, plus the usual array of school events. Believe me, the expression "never a dull moment" certainly applied to our household!

In 2001, Hélène and I decided to move our little family to another suburb just to the east of Toronto. Shortly afterwards, I was recruited through a head-hunter by a local company for a top management position and began with them in January of 2002. I was now living ten minutes from my work. Although I had regretfully given up my regular tennis games, I was now pursuing a superior leisure passion – music. I was playing lead guitar in a little classic rock band and we actually played a few gigs in some of the local pubs and even in one little place near downtown Toronto in an area known as the Beaches. Life was good! Life was fulfilling! And so much fun!

My life is so different now. Each waking moment includes a painful, mind-twisting exercise that I just wish could be over. Every day, my brain takes me through the moment by moment routines that we all do and tend to take for granted. I can no longer walk. My left leg and foot are paralyzed and are painfully stiff. My left arm is totally numb and my left hand and fingers are tightly clenched and I experience a severe stinging sensation all the time. I suppose you could say that it sometimes appears as though I have gotten used to it but when I do stop and think about this affliction, it is just heartbreaking. The left side of my face is always numb and my lips and pronunciation seem to drag. Also, I usually gnaw at the inside of my cheek.

Today, I am driving with my family to the Ottawa Valley to see my Dad, my sister, her daughter and a couple of my Dad's sisters (my aunts). As I sit in my spot in the front passenger seat of our Venture van, I am daydreaming and thinking about my youth beyond 20 years, which now happens to be about 27 years ago.

Why the hell did I have to have this stroke thingy? I was enjoying life and my activities so much. Four days before this "brain attack" I was enjoying performing a great night of rock music with Tom and some other great musicians. Man, did we rock! It was an awesome time.

CHAPTER 2:   DAY-TO-DAY LIFE

I read the news today, Oh Boy,
About a lucky man...

So let me share a bit more with you about what initially happened to me when I had my first stroke and then some of what my new life and typical day-to-day routine are like now.

Before I had my stroke, I was a pretty happy and balanced guy, living with my two boys, Corey and Tyler and my then common-law wife, Hélène, who is now my exquisitely 'legal' wife. Each day, I would get up to get ready for work and, on the way to the kitchen for some cottage cheese and berries and a glass of milk, I would pick up my guitar from its stand in the corner of our bedroom, carry it downstairs to our living room and play a few chords for a minute or two of a few songs I had rehearsed the night before. Then I would smile as I thought about my band partners, Tom, Wayne and Art and our plans to perform together at a local pub in a couple of days. We had made plans for our band to play with the normally booked guys and hopefully get our other "Hilroy" band members together to play some of the original stuff we had developed as well as some of the incredible cover songs we had learned to play so well.

Day-to-day life was usually pretty hectic and I always had something fresh and interesting to which I could look forward. Fortunately, we had moved to a town where my place of work was only ten minutes away, so my commute was a fraction of what it had been for several years. Our band usually tried to practice a couple of nights a week and, initially, most practices were held in Wayne's basement, as it was easier for Tom, Art and I to move our relatively portable electronic equipment than it would have been for Wayne to move his drum kit.

Quite often, by the time I got home it was 11:30 pm or later. Unfortunately, there was still office work waiting for me and I usually got on my laptop at that God awful hour and plugged away for at least a couple of hours. My alarm clock usually went off at 6 or 6:30 am, which quite often left me feeling as though I really hadn't had much sleep at all!

In retrospect, between my high blood pressure, the lack of exercise (remember, I had given up tennis when we moved east of Toronto), the pressures of my job as well as the long hours it demanded, plus the usual stress associated with running a household, I was actually a stroke or heart attack looking for a place to happen! The morning the shit hit the fan, so to speak, Hélène remembers her mother telling her that "life as you know it will never be the same". Man, was she ever right!

Now, some three years later, a typical day for Hélène and me starts the way a usual evening ends. A typical evening usually ends with me lying peacefully in bed with my adoring, beautiful wife close beside me and with us appreciating each other and winding down from a hectic and busy appointment-filled day. My wife and I enjoy each other's company so much that a person should be able to market and sell what we have. We are very happy with what we have and share together.

On most weekends, we try to have a little time for ourselves and we might take any combination of the boys or all of them out with us for dinner, go to a movie by ourselves or go with our friends Tom and Janet or Dale and Bonnie.

Every day, my fingers and toes tingle like bee stings and the bottom of my feet ache despite and because of the prevailing paralysis I have on my left side. Of course, my stroke and the resulting paralysis has left my entire left side non-functional and penetrated with Thalamic Pain 24/7 (look it up on the Internet). At any particular moment, I do not have any pain or uncomfortable sensations in my limbs but my extremities are tingling with pain all the time. Whenever the tingling settles in, we make sure that I take a couple of tabs of an amazingly effective pain medication called Lyrica during the course of any evening. Lyrica seems to be the answer to most of the discomfort I get but it certainly provides a rather soothing and relatively euphoric 'high' state that seems to settle a lot of my discomfort. My usual daily serving of prescriptions and their dosages and purposes includes the following:

Name	Dose	Purpose
NORVASC	1 x 10 mg tab/day	blood pressure
LABETALOL	3 x 100 mg tabs/day	blood pressure
ALTACE	1 x 10 mg tab/day	blood pressure
HYDROCHLOROTHIAZIDE	1 x 12.5 mg tab/day	blood pressure
BACLOFEN	2 x 10 mg tabs/day	spasticity

LYRICA	2 x 75 mg tabs/day	pain
CRANBERRY	2 x 9000 mg tabs/day	prevent U.T.I.*
B COMPLEX	1 20 mg tab/day	nerve regeneration
DIDROCAL	1 500 mg tab/day	calcium supplement
BUSPAR	2 x 10 mg tabs/day	anti-depressant
ELAVIL	2 x 10 mg tabs/day	nerve pain
RANITIDINE	1 x 150 mg	antacid
TEMAZEPAM	1 x 30 mg	sleep aid

*Urinary Tract Infection

… A virtual pharmacy wouldn't you say?

I can confidently say that I almost always have a perfectly sound and restful sleep, but I have been known to occasionally wake up anywhere between 4:00 and 8:00 am and wheel over to the computer room and work on my book on our computer. I am sorry to say that Hélène does not always get that much deserved and badly needed complete night's sleep because, unfortunately, I sometimes snore and wake her up. In those cases, she normally quietly slides out of our bed to sleep on the day bed in the computer room, unnoticed by me. If my mind should waken me with a thought or an idea that occurs to me as potentially interesting or possibly pertinent to any of the themes I am developing for my book, I will get up and spend one to three or four hours on my manuscript which is progressing nicely, currently at more than 85k words. My goal is to get it into the hands of an interested publisher within the next few weeks.

A typical day, from my perspective, starts when I wake up, usually between 7:00 and 8:00 am. However, today has been one of those mornings when I have woken and gone to the computer room at 5:00 am and typed out about three or four more pages for my book. As I work, I gradually become aware once more of the never ending pain in my fingers and toes and I simply close out the relentless sensations and I continue with my focus on my writing, totally disregarding the pain in my fingers and toes and the pressure in my head (for more information and background on "How I Feel", refer to A STROKE SURVIVOR'S JOURNAL – HOW I FEEL in the Appendix).

I usually work away uninterrupted until about 8:00 am when Corey's alarm goes off. He gets up without hesitation and has breakfast, watches about 20 minutes of TV, chats with me for a few minutes and without fail, is always dressed and ready and heading out the door at 8:30 am for his 15 minute brisk jog to school. At about that time, I hear Hélène rousing from her night's sleep and a few minutes later, she appears at the computer room door and walks over to deposit her 'good morning' kiss.

I close off whatever work I had open on the PC and a typical new day has started. Fifteen minutes later, the scheduled personal care worker arrives at the door, lets him or herself in by entering his or her assigned security code to the front door lock and prepares the bathtub area for my daily shower and makes the bed. We have this personal service for me, provided by the government, as warranted by my disability. I speak elsewhere in this book (see "Routines", Section 6, Chapter 2) of the wonderful people who are part of an ever revolving chain of personal care providers who parade through our home on a 'seven days a week' basis. We also have a housekeeper who comes in once a week to clean house and who basically helps Hélène keep up with her housekeeping and miscellaneous chores and errands. Christine is usually in at 10:00 am and out by 1:00 pm. Susan, this particular day's personal service provider, who may be one of three or four PSWs who are part of the service, helps me dress and prepares me for my day. She prepares and brings me my breakfast, makes our bed, cleans the bathroom and usually heads out the door with us as we get in to the car to drive to any one of a range of daily appointments. Susan then drives on to her next client. A typical day for us involves Hélène getting me into the car and driving us around our quaint little town to any of a few destinations including my acupuncturist, my family doctor, my physiatrist, my neurologist, either of two of our usual pharmacies and any other retail destination that we have to run our errands at this day. PHEW! Do you get my drift?

So, an evening ends at about midnight for Hélène and me as we quietly watch the last moments of any particular show that happens to be running at the end of our viewing day. Corey always disappears off to bed promptly at 11:00 on any school night. Almost always, we both nod off for the night together by 12:00 or 12:30 am and enjoy a sound sleep. Most evenings, we go to bed together at any time between 8:00 and 9:00 pm and relax in front of the television set which is about seven feet from the floor on top of the wall unit sitting on top of Hélène's dresser, positioned along the wall at the foot of our bed. Each weekday night, we select from a range of our favorite shows available on the digital cable service to which we subscribe. The show we watch could be any of our usual shows: "CSI", "American Idol", "24", "Without a Trace" or "Crossing Jordan".

Occasionally, Corey will join us in our room to watch a show and will usually sit in my wheelchair while Hélène and I cozy up together in our bed. Most other nights, Corey will settle in front of our huge, 42", hi-definition, Sony Vega television set in our family room downstairs and watch any of his favorite shows or he will get on his drum kit and practice a really cool drum riff or whatever he was learning in his drum lessons that particular week.

Our evenings are quiet, calm, relaxing and comfortable. Hélène and I soothe each other with kind, affectionate words and the occasional peck on the cheek or lips and Hélène prepares and gives me my scheduled medication for that particular night. The evening may be fragmented by some humor and, of course, we may erupt into a typical family discussion about Corey's day at school or he might entertain us with an interesting description about how any of his numerous snow-boarding trips have gone this week. Corey has a season pass at the Lakeridge ski hill, just 20 minutes from our home and he has gone about three or four times so far this winter on significant ski trips in the surrounding areas. What a perfect winter it has been for snow-boarders; lots of snow and not too cold!

I suppose this description of a typical evening for us sounds like any you might have and you could probably compare much of it with your own. Unfortunately, a typical evening for us is not that normal as any time spent like this is usually comprised of considerable pain and discomfort for me. However, we all do enjoy our peaceful evenings and consider ourselves lucky to have what we do have. Our youngest son, who still lives with us, is in our thoughts, plans and concerns at every waking moment. We also worry and think about our middle son, Tyler, who also still has a few miles to travel. We have recently celebrated his success at getting his high school diploma. We are so proud! Now, his next obvious required step is to find himself a half decent job and possibly get some post-secondary education. We will be there for him whatever he plans to do. He is a smart and personable young man. He will do well, of that we are certain.

The eldest, Paul, fortunately is right where he needs to be right now. He is living in British Columbia with his girlfriend, Colleen. They are both working at the same hotel right now. We hope to find the right timing to be able to visit them some time in the next few months. We'll see...

CHAPTER 3: LOUD MOUTH LOUIE'S

It was Thursday, February 13th. Tom and I had arranged to meet at Loud Mouth Louie's on Queen Street in the Beaches to perform some blues and classic rock music with a few guys that we had met just a few weeks before and played with a few times. We had all jammed together the previous Thursday.

I brought my Eric Clapton Stratocaster, "Blackie", and my powerful and loud Fender "Chorus" Amp. I also brought my "Wah" and my distortion pedals. Altogether, our equipment made phenomenal sounds. Tom had taught me how to perform comfortably in front of an audience and I had developed considerable confidence and guitar skills, or so I was repeatedly told by friends and colleagues.

At about 9:00 pm that night, our musician friends set up their equipment and turned on their amps. Tom is the most amazing and natural keyboardist you could want to play with and listen to. At practices, he had always impressed me and he knew an endless list of the best "classic rock" tunes. Tom and I had put together a long list of great classic rock songs with which we were familiar and were prepared to play. Our regular bassist, Art, and our drummer, Wayne, weren't available that night, but our new musician friends were happy to play with us and we prepared to perform an evening of the greatest classic rock tunes. That night, WE ROCKED!!

I have to say that, yes, I was a little nervous at first, in fact, I was excited that we were about to perform. Hélène had invited a couple of our friends from her work and the three of them were comfortably settled in for a night of cold ales and good tunes. I usually had my music songbook binder with me, complete with the lyrics and the chords of a huge collection of popular songs. At around 9:30 pm, we struck up the first notes of Eric Clapton's "Cocaine" and our friends and the other patrons in the pub were clearly pleased and impressed with the sound. Tom and I smiled at each other, as usual, and we also smiled appreciatively at our new musician partners. We were creating a magical sound. I was in another world! I was so grateful of this experience.

We were pleased with the artistic cooperation and resulting successful output. Upon proceeding getting about 30% through the tune, Tom and I jointly keyed through some outstanding lead breaks and I fretted some amazing guitar solos. We then rocked to Neil Young's "Helpless" and Santana's "Black Magic Woman" and some famous Beatles' tunes among a few others.

At about 11:30 pm, Hélène said she needed to go home, as her work day started at 7:00 am. As she had joined us at the pub in her own car and Tom and I came in my van, she was able to leave ahead of us. Tom and I continued playing until about 1:00 am, when we eventually packed our equipment into the van and headed home. It had been a magical evening.

Four days later, I had my stroke which unfortunately meant the end of any continued promise with my guitar. It was heartbreaking to say the least. Hélène had the unpleasant task of telling Tom and the other musicians that I was totally out of commission and looking like I would not be returning to the stage any time soon.

SECTION FOUR – IF ONLY I HAD KNOWN

CHAPTER 1: I SHOULD HAVE KNOWN BETTER

About two weeks or so before the first of my two strokes, I started experiencing blinding headaches. No amount of Tylenol would provide relief. I had rarely suffered from headaches in the past and consequently, I never put two and two together. I had attempted to make an appointment to see my family physician, but unfortunately he was fully booked that day and couldn't fit me in. All I could do for the time being was grin and bear it.

On February 11th, six days prior to my first stroke, I had an appointment at the hospital for routine tests as part of my annual physical. My G.P. then was affiliated with a hospital that was about an hour's drive from our home. By the time I arrived there for the tests, my blood pressure was "through the roof" and any tests were out of the question until it had stabilized. I was sent to the Emergency Department and, as we all know, the wait in such a place can be interminable. After lying on a gurney for three or four hours, a resident examined me and indicated that my blood pressure had begun to subside and, given the distance between the hospital and my home, he would not be admitting me. He assured me that it would be safe for me to go home. He prescribed a second blood pressure medication and stipulated that I was to visit my family physician before the end of the week, which I did do two days later to make sure. When I got there, my blood pressure was still reading high, so he increased the dose of the new medication and told me to come back on Tuesday. Unfortunately, I would never make it.

After my "last performance" at Loud Mouth Louie's that night, I had a short good night's sleep and, before I knew it, it was once more time to go to work. It was Valentine's Day and Hélène and I had made plans to go out for a romantic dinner that evening. However, when Hélène got home from work, she found me asleep in bed! I told her I was very tired and didn't feel well enough to go out. We decided to celebrate Valentine's Day the next night instead. The weekend was quiet. I still wasn't feeling the best, so we spent the weekend just doing some quiet things around the house. Little did we know, but I should have been admitting myself to hospital, thereby avoiding this debilitating, life-threatening nightmare! My head had probably started bleeding a few days earlier. How was one to know?

I had finally gotten rid of my headache, so we went out to dinner on Saturday night and had a very nice time at a restaurant a few blocks away that we had seen but to which we had never been as yet called "Krebs". The food was great, the service was excellent and we were extremely well received, especially considering we didn't even have a reservation – on Valentine's Day weekend, the busiest weekend of the year for a restaurant! Gary and Patricia, you and your staff are the best and you deserve the success you are now reaping! In fact, we were so impressed that night that "Krebs" would one day play a crucial part in the most special day of our lives…

On Monday morning, I got up for work, feeling quite normal and went to use the bathroom. I had asked Hélène to get me up early as I had to drive a couple of hours to

Cambridge that day for a series of business meetings. As I began to get dressed, I suddenly felt a tingling in my left leg and the next thing I knew I was on the floor and could not get up. Hélène appeared at that moment and asked me what I was doing down there! I was conscious and I asked her to help me get up, which she attempted to do. When I told her what had happened and what I had felt, she suspected immediately that I had had a stroke and quickly dialed 9-1-1. The paramedics arrived within about ten minutes and, after checking my vital signs and asking me a few questions, they bundled me on to the gurney. Our two youngest boys were still at home that morning while all this was happening and Hélène went and woke them up so they wouldn't be alarmed by the paramedics, the ambulance and all the commotion. As this was all happening at around 6:00 am on the 17th of February, the temperature outside was well below zero and I still remember thinking how warm my bed had been only a few minutes earlier! Some of the neighbours who were heading off to work noticed the unusual activity at the Frost household and were naturally curious. No time for chit-chat that morning though! Soon the ambulance was speeding down Highway 2 towards Ajax-Pickering Hospital, with Hélène and the boys following closely behind.

After spending several hours in the Emergency Department, a CT scan revealed that I'd had a hemorrhagic bleed between the lobes of the brain and that, because any intervention would lead to more bleeding, it was inoperable. There was also some evidence of hydrocephalus or water on the brain. The Internist who took over my case told Hélène that we would have to wait for the blood to be re-absorbed into my brain and to be prepared that my recovery would be a long, slow one.

It was determined at the hospital that, having had one stroke, there was also significant risk of yet another one. Imagine that, healthy and mobile one moment and near death and paralyzed the next, and not even in a car accident!

I spent the next couple of days in Intensive Care, unable to eat or drink because of the paralysis on the left side of my face and in my throat. Hélène and the boys still laugh about my obsession with "Fruit Explosion Muffins" from Tim Horton's! That's all I kept asking for, day after day. The nurses there were always extremely attentive, caring and supportive to Hélène and the boys as they waited patiently for my condition to improve. That was so crucial.

I was moved into a semi-private room on Wednesday, sharing with a young man who had accidentally suffered chemical poisoning at his work 10 years before. He couldn't breathe without a breathing tube and, as a result, could not speak other than to use hand signals and moans and groans to keep telling all the ladies (including Hélène) how pretty they were! The first night I was in the room with him (unfortunately, I don't remember his name), he was rushed back to Intensive Care because of a sudden problem he was having with his breathing. I wouldn't see him again until three weeks later.

CHAPTER 2:   CODE BLUE

The next few weeks were an absolute nightmare as I was in and out of consciousness and even had a "Code Blue" (cardiac arrest) called on me on at least one occasion. Slipping in and out of consciousness, I had many strange dreams, the kind one would hear about on an episode of The Twilight Zone.

At first, I was very much aware of the strange, new environment at the Ajax-Pickering Hospital. It was all very confusing, made even more so by the fact that my short-term memory was affected right from day one. Hélène was with me every day and I had the occasional visitor, although the doctors had asked that visiting be curtailed, other than immediate family, until they could get my blood pressure under control. I usually drifted in and out of a deep sleep each day and Hélène tells me that I went through a delusional period where I was seeing bugs on the walls and people "flying" outside in front of my window! After a couple of months had passed, I didn't really remember much of what had happened throughout this whole experience. Even for months after I first recovered from my initial attack, I did not clearly remember or understand what had happened.

One thing I did know was that Hélène had always been my best friend and, as only best friends will do, she stayed by my side throughout my ordeal. One day, about a week after my stroke, I lay in my hospital bed, unable to sleep. I knew in my heart what had to be done. I then buzzed the nurse to help me dial my home phone number. It was 5:45 am. As Hélène was still very worried about me, she answered the phone on the first ring. When I heard her voice, I told her that I had decided what we needed to do. I then asked her to marry me. We had been best friends and wonderful partners for six years already and I just couldn't imagine being without her. Though she had been hoping for the prospect of our getting married for quite a while, the actual proposal came as a complete surprise to her. She accepted immediately and, excitedly, we began talking about the wedding and making plans. We even talked about going down to the Bahamas to get married on the beach. We have been there before and we both love the islands. In the midst of a rather uncertain medical situation, it gave us something positive and exciting to which we could look forward.

However, our plans abruptly took a back seat at the end of that week. As I was beginning to recuperate, I had another hemorrhagic bleed which put me out of commission once more. This one was much more serious as it was located in the cerebellum or brain stem. Too much blood in this area could have quickly led to my death. In addition, there was, once again, evidence of hydrocephalus. This condition was putting considerable pressure on my brain and was actually shifting it to one side of my skull. The accumulation of blood would have to be removed immediately or I would not live through the weekend.

An ambulance arrived within minutes to transport me to Toronto Western Hospital. Tyler and Corey had arrived just as the paramedics were wheeling me out of my room and I know they were very frightened by the scene they were witnessing. At least they were able to see me before I left. It was 5:50 pm on Friday, February 28th.

Anyone who lives in or around Toronto knows that Friday night on the Don Valley Parkway (or the Don Valley parking lot, as we affectionately call it) is a nightmare. By the time the paramedics loaded my gurney into the bus and the nurse who accompanied me as well as Hélène and the two paramedics were safely in the ambulance, we left Ajax at 6:00 pm or so, sirens blaring and lights flashing! We drove for about 20 minutes or so, dodging traffic. Fortunately, other drivers around us were courteous and moved out of our way when they saw the lights and heard the siren, but it was still taking too long to get there in a reasonable time and we still had a long way to go. Then suddenly the paramedic who was riding with me in the back noticed a police car coming up behind us. He called out to the ambulance driver to let the officer get by so we could follow him. This is exactly what we did, driving on the shoulder of the DVP until we reached our exit ramp. We arrived at Toronto Western by about 6:50 pm

A team of doctors was waiting for us in the Emergency Room and they quickly prepped me for surgery. They asked Hélène several key questions about my medical background and took my vital signs. The anesthetist asked Hélène what they needed to know and Hélène informed her that I was/am a hemophiliac. Although I squeezed Hélène's hand and responded that this was an "insignificant" condition, the anesthetist disagreed with this dismissive response and was fortunately able to have a few bags of the appropriate blood plasma ready for me, should the need arise. As it turns out, surgery took 4 ½ hours instead of the anticipated two or three and I was given four units of blood. The surgery, fortunately, was a complete success. The neurosurgeon had removed the accumulating blood and inserted a "shunt" which would drain the excess fluid from my brain.

I should mention here that my relatively minor hemophilia had been discovered when I was a child and had had a tooth pulled. Throughout my life, this poor blood clotting condition had never been a real problem. My typical minor cuts and gashes always healed immediately, hence my perception that it was "insignificant"!

When I was about 14 years old, I had to have a molar removed. It was quite a harrowing experience. My dentist at the time had not yet adopted an oral hygiene program in his practice. In fact, oral hygiene was not a standard process that most dentists made a practice of offering in those days. The solution to any decay discovered in a tooth was to just pull it out!

My poor Dad had been born with soft teeth and unfortunately it looked like I had inherited the soft tooth trait as well because every time I went to the dentist I had to have a couple of fillings. It seemed like I had gotten used to the extensive restorative dental work required at each of my appointments. Fortunately for me, Mom and Dad were quite worried about my retaining my teeth, I suppose because of Dad's experience and they made sure I made frequent trips to have my teeth cleaned, polished and filled.

Also, fortunately, dentists were just starting to include oral hygiene and fluoride as a regular part of their routines when examining and repairing teeth. I remember, one time when I had gone for a check up at only 12 years of age, my dentist discovered a major cavity and decided to pull the tooth. He pulled it, resulting in extensive and prolonged bleeding. I remember that my Mom had put me to bed with a bowl for me to frequently spit out all the blood that was collecting in my cheeks. It was so gross. I would spit out gobs of blood. Because of a condition I had of hemophilia, huge pockets of blood were accumulating inside my mouth and the wound just wouldn't quite heal immediately or actually stop bleeding. So much blood would accumulate without totally coagulating that it would collect in my throat, eventually causing me to vomit. At times, I would spit up so much blood that it would project across the room (a la Linda Blair). My poor Mom had to keep up with the mess. Somehow, she saw me through the experience and I managed to remain healthy all through my adolescence.

Mom and Dad made an appointment for me to see a specialist in Montréal about this condition. It was concluded that I was a hemophiliac with just a 10% deficiency in Factor 8, a significant clotting agent of the blood. In subsequent years, I experienced a stable and normal childhood, youth and growth into maturity, without any further bleeding incidents.

Like most kids, I did occasionally cut or gash my foot and it always healed fairly quickly and normally, thank God. Time went by and, when I was about 23 years old, I went to a specialist near my home in Ottawa. The knowledgeable doctor conducted an extensive series of tests and again determined that I had a minor clotting deficiency. There was no concern raised at the time, but little did I know that this condition would eventually contribute to the complications I had during my hemorrhagic bleed, the cause of my stroke! We're not aware that the hemophilia actually played any part in causing my stroke but only that it contributed to the bleeding continuing once it had started.

Anyway, the good doctors were able to get the bleeding under control with customary blood products and soon the pressure was relieved and the critical condition was normalized.

I spent the next two weeks at Toronto Western Hospital, the first few days in the Intensive Care Unit, then to the Step-Down Unit and, finally, in a semi-private room on the medical floor. After two weeks, the doctors at Western determined that they had done everything they could for me neurologically and that it was time for me to go back to my community hospital, Ajax-Pickering.

I arrived back on a Friday afternoon in March (to the same room and the same roommate I had left two weeks prior) and was slowly but surely re-introduced to semi-solid foods (up to that point I had been fed liquids through a tube in my nose!). Hélène had gone back to work that week, but had adjusted her hours so she could be at the hospital by 3:00 pm. On the Tuesday following my return to Ajax-Pickering, Hélène arrived at the hospital to find a team of medical professionals surrounding my hospital bed. As she tells it now, having spent the previous two weeks visiting me in a "teaching hospital", her immediate thought was that Ajax-Pickering had now become one as well. Little did she know!

One of the nurses, who had gotten to know us well, approached Hélène as she stood in the doorway of my room and told her that she had been trying to reach her on her cell phone. They had apparently just missed each other, as Hélène had turned her phone off as she entered the hospital. The nurse suggested that Hélène accompany her to the ICU lounge to talk. Hélène knew immediately that there was a problem and she became understandably agitated. She eventually agreed to go to the lounge where the nurse and a social worker explained to her that they had called a "Code Blue" (cardiac arrest) on me. They did explain that my heart had never actually stopped but that my pulse and my blood pressure had become so low that it was decided not to wait until my heart actually did stop. Better to have everyone there beforehand. At that point, my blood pressure was extremely low (80/60 - remember that what put me in the hospital in the first place was high blood pressure!) and I was totally unresponsive, so a decision was made to transfer me into the Intensive Care Unit for closer observation. It was thought that I was probably suffering from pneumonia for the second time since my first stroke but, quite honestly, they weren't quite sure what was happening. They even did a spinal tap, thinking it might be meningitis. After a few weeks, the results of the spinal tap came back negative and we never did find out what had caused my sudden "crash".

While Hélène was waiting to see me, she had attempted to contact my brother Brian at his work. Unfortunately, he was on a First Aid course that day and could not be reached. So, Hélène was forced to wait (and worry) by herself. At about 4:30 pm or so, Brian arrived at the hospital and Hélène immediately informed him of what had happened. Together they waited to see me and talk to the doctor. When they were finally able to come into the ICU, they were informed that my blood pressure was still low, that they were doing everything possible to raise it (within reason, of course) and that they would monitor me very closely. Whenever there is a problem with blood pressure, the key is to lower it (or raise it, whichever the case may be) in a controlled way – i.e. not too quickly – as any sudden change can bring on a seizure. I was hooked up to a blood pressure monitor, which made it somewhat easier to keep an eye on my condition. Once it was clear that my blood pressure was increasing comfortably, at about 8:30 pm or so Hélène and Brian both left the hospital and headed home, but not until Hélène had extracted a promise from my nurse that she would call her at home no matter what if anything happened.

At 10:00 pm, Hélène was tucking our youngest, Corey, into bed and explaining to him what had happened to me. She had promised our boys from day one of our crisis that, no matter what, she would not keep anything from them regarding my condition. So, as she was tending to Corey, the phone rang. It was the ICU nurse who was watching over me that night. She told Hélène that my blood pressure had dropped again, that I was becoming less and less responsive and that she had sent me down to Diagnostic Imaging for a CT scan. She also indicated that they would probably need to intubate me and put me on a respirator. She suggested that perhaps Hélène would like to be there when I came back up to the floor. Hélène immediately called my brother, who lived just up the street from us, and they agreed to meet at the hospital. Understandably, I apparently wasn't too thrilled with the breathing tube, according to Hélène! Whenever I was awake, I would cough because this thing was down my throat and then I would choke, with no sound coming out. She says to this day that watching me struggle with the tube was one of the most difficult things she has ever had to watch. She felt very helpless. Mercifully, the doctors kept me sedated that night so I wouldn't struggle with the tube. Hélène stayed with me until about 1:00 am and then went home to get some much needed rest. Who knew what tomorrow would bring?

The next morning, Hélène met with my attending physician, Doctor Baker, who admitted that, in retrospect, the hospital never should have taken me back as they were not equipped to handle the complexity of my case, having neither a hematology department nor a neurologist on staff. As a result, every time there was blood taken from me for analysis, it was sent by cab to a downtown hospital. By the time the results came back, my condition had changed again, so erratic was my "roller-coaster ride".

The doctor indicated to Hélène that they had put out a "Criti-Call", which is a province-wide alert to all hospitals that had a neurologist on staff, a hematology department and an available bed. She said that I could be transferred anywhere in the province and prepared Hélène for the possibility that I might not end up at a local hospital. All they could do then was wait and pray.

CHAPTER 3:   CRITI-CALL

Luckily, it took only a few hours for us to get a response to the "Criti-Call" and, for once, it was good news! I was going to Mt. Sinai Hospital in Toronto! Even the Internist who had been overseeing my case at Ajax-Pickering was thrilled when he learned the news. I couldn't have been going to a better place, as far as he was concerned. In fact, his roommate from Medical School would be my attending physician.

On the afternoon of March 19th, the ambulance arrived to transfer me downtown. Just before I left, my brother's girlfriend picked Tyler and Corey up at home and brought them to the hospital to see me. I was completely out of it, of course, but it made them feel better to see me for a few minutes.

When we arrived at Mt. Sinai, I was taken up to the 18th floor Intensive Care Unit, where a team of doctors and nurses was waiting for me. I was pretty much out of it but I know Hélène and Brian were relieved to see me in such a wonderful place.

The next morning, Hélène arrived to see me and was surprised to find me sitting up in bed, minus the breathing tube, smiling and waving to her! I even said "Hi, honey" in a somewhat raspy voice. Imagine her surprise (and relief)! I had a nurse who was dedicated exclusively to my care and I was being monitored closely. As visiting hours were basically 24/7, Hélène could stay with me as long as she wanted.

As the next few days passed, my condition changed continuously, sometimes from one hour to the next. It was somewhat disconcerting for my family, needless to say, as they really didn't know what to expect. Hélène visited me every day and was there from 11:00 am until 7:00 or 8:00 pm, with a short break for lunch. Once she got home, she would make phone calls to my Mom and Dad, my sister, my brother, as well as our many friends who had called and left messages (sometimes as many as 9 or 10 in one night!!), filling them in on my condition and the events of that day, including whatever the doctors had told her. Then she would try to grab a bite to eat and spend some quality time with Tyler and Corey. Unfortunately, Paul had left for a long ago planned trip to Hawaii shortly after my first stroke and was scheduled to be away for six months!

This was the pattern of our life for the next week or so… then all hell broke loose!

CHAPTER 4: WHAT IN THE WORLD IS S.A.R.S.?

About a week after my arrival at Mt. Sinai, the media started reporting about something called S.A.R.S. Of course, I knew nothing of this as I was sleeping away most of my days and was blissfully unaware of what was going on in the outside world.

It was the night before my 50th birthday. Brian and his girlfriend dropped by to see me. I don't remember their visit, but have been told this is what happened. Anyway, they knew they wouldn't be able to come by on my actual birthday due to a scheduling conflict, so they made the trip after work the day prior. Little did they know that would be the last time they would see me for several weeks!

The next day, my big 5 – 0, Hélène was with me all day. A week earlier, she had sent an email to all our friends and relatives, updating them on my condition. She had told them that my 50th was coming up and asked those who were interested to please send birthday wishes that she could then read to me in the hospital. She printed off the ones we received by email and brought them to me, along with the cards I had received over the past few days. She read some of them to me, but I got tired and she had to stop. When she arrived at the hospital that morning, she wished me a HAPPY BIRTHDAY and gave me a kiss. She then said "I'll bet you can think of better ways to spend your 50th birthday!" and I said "THAT'S FOR SURE!!" According to Hélène, it was actually one of the only clear things I said all day.

Around mid-afternoon, when Hélène was in the visitors' lounge making a phone call to the boys, the social worker for the ICU dropped by to see her. She had the unfortunate task of informing Hélène and the other visitors to the ICU that the S.A.R.S. outbreak, which had been reported on the news and in the newspapers for the past few days, was now critical and that the hospital was being forced to curtail all visitors. On Sunday night, a patient had been transferred into the ICU at Mt. Sinai from Scarborough Grace Hospital. As the S.A.R.S. epidemic had started at Scarborough Grace, it had been virtually shut down. The gentleman in question was at Mt. Sinai until Tuesday morning and was on the opposite side of the unit from where I was. They didn't even know whether this person had been exposed to the illness, but they weren't taking any chances. They shut down the ICU - no new patients coming in and none transferring out.

After the initial shock (and many tears), Hélène was told to stay with me as long as she could that day and then to go home and wait for more news.

Although they had initially said "No visitors", they finally realized that they needed to be somewhat lenient and decided to allow one family member to go in, if absolutely necessary. Obviously, in our case it WAS absolutely necessary! That same visitor was the only one who could come in on any given day. This, of course, meant that neither the boys nor my brother would be allowed in to see me. Needless to say, they were all disappointed and would need to rely even more on Hélène and her daily updates.

So, while Hélène took the day after my birthday off (the first time in three weeks), she was right back by my side again the next day. On a daily basis, she would go through the screening process, answering a multitude of questions and getting her temperature taken. She had to wear goggles, a mask, a gown and gloves before going anywhere near the unit. Not much fun, but better than just staying home and wondering how I was doing.

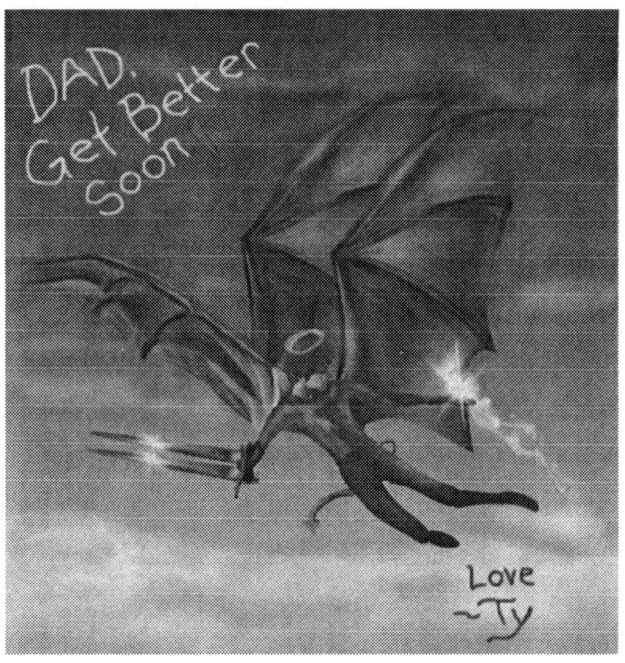

A creation by my son, Tyler

A few days after the visiting restrictions were imposed, on a Sunday morning in late March, Hélène was walking onto the GO train to head down to spend the day with me when her cell phone rang. It was Margaret, my day shift nurse. She asked Hélène how far away she was from the hospital and encouraged her to get to the hospital as quickly as possible. Margaret said I had taken a turn for the worse, my temperature having soared to 41º Celsius or 105º Fahrenheit!!

I was delirious at this point and my blood pressure was up in the 200s! The doctor then got on the phone with Hélène. He said it was possible that I had had another stroke, but nothing could be confirmed without an MRI (Magnetic Resonance Imaging). He asked Hélène whether I had any metal in my body (plate, etc.) and she said no, not to her knowledge (and I can tell you now that I didn't). He told her to get there as soon as possible but not to panic – I was in good hands.

When Hélène arrived in the ICU, after the usual screening which, of course, seemed to take forever that day, she discovered that my temperature had gone down a bit (to 39º C or 102º F), thanks to Margaret's resourcefulness! She had packed me in ice from head to toe!

A decision had been made to perform a CT scan, rather than an MRI. However, there was a problem. In order to seal off the ICU from visitors during the S.A.R.S. crisis, the power source to the automatic double doors had been turned off, which meant they couldn't get me (in my hospital bed) to the bank of elevators. Only one door could be opened manually and the other one was locked. The bed wouldn't fit through the door! After about 30 minutes of attempting to open the second door and trying to call a service man up to unlock it, one of the PSWs discovered that the freight elevator was unlocked and that my bed would fit in it. So, down we went… Margaret, two PSWs, a security guard, Hélène and me in my bed on a stinky old garbage elevator! Necessity is the mother of invention, as they say! We arrived at Diagnostic Imaging and the technician was waiting for us, having been called in from home as all services in the hospital had been cancelled because of the emergency situation in the city. He took me into the X-Ray room while the others waited in the hallway. The CT scan showed no change from the previous one, a good thing apparently. Unfortunately, the doctor still had no idea what had caused my fever. One of those good news/bad news situations, I guess! At least I hadn't had another stroke! They never did figure out what had happened.

A few days later, after watching me pull my feeding tube out of my nose three or four times (in one day!), the doctor suggested that I have a G-tube inserted. The "G" stands for gastro-intestinal. The insertion of the tube required a small incision in my stomach. Again, Hélène accompanied me downstairs. After the surgeon had explained everything to her, including the slight danger in any procedure, Hélène signed the release form and off I went. The procedure only took a few minutes and, before I knew it, I was back in my room in the ICU (when my high fever episode occurred, Margaret had arranged to move me into a small private room within the ICU). I had that G-tube in until May sometime, when it was accidentally pulled out when I was being transferred from my bed into my wheelchair. By then, I had started eating semi-solid food. But more on that later…

After about two weeks or so, the doctors indicated that I was ready to be moved to the Step-Down Unit two floors below. Another one of those good news/bad news situations. The good news was that I had improved enough for them to consider me off the critical list and able to move on to the next step; the bad news was that there were NO VISITORS (and that included Hélène) in the SDU!! She tried everything she could think of to get them to change their minds…Nothing doing! They did, however, tell her she could go into the SDU with me when I was transferred and she did exactly that. They even told her that she could stay as long as she wanted, which is exactly what she did.

Unfortunately, this would be the last time we would see each other for almost five weeks!

SECTION FIVE – A NEW LIFE

CHAPTER 1: HERE, THERE AND EVERYWHERE

Over the next few days, Hélène noticed (and it was confirmed by the nurses) that I seemed to be very confused. I talked to her on the phone about...going on the bus...going for a boat ride...living in Alta Vista (that's in Ottawa, for the uninitiated)...all told, I was quite mixed up. Needless to say, I asked her constantly when she was coming to pick me up (at one point, I even asked when she was going to be home, that I was waiting for her!). The worse part was that there didn't seem to be an end in sight. In fact, the doctor told Hélène one night that it was possible she wouldn't be able to see me until I was transferred to a long-term rehab facility! When she said this, Hélène's immediate reaction was "But that could take weeks!" to which the doctor replied "That's right!" The doctor was obviously preparing Hélène for the worst case scenario.

As frustrating as it all was, it was more frustrating to know that I was asking the nurses why Hélène didn't want to come and see me anymore! That broke her heart! Needless to say, the nurses then reassured me that that was not the case.

Eventually, I was moved to a regular room (private because of S.A.R.S.), which I guess was a good sign. Obviously, I must have been getting better, if they were willing to let me out of the Step-Down Unit. At one point, they actually started talking about moving me to a Stroke Rehab facility (there are four of them in the GTA), although I wasn't quite ready for that yet. But soon, we hoped!

On Thursday, May 8th, 2003, I had the most wonderful surprise! The social worker on the medical/surgical floor called Hélène at home and informed her that I was being moved to Bridgepoint Health, a long-term rehab facility in Toronto. She also told my wife that she would be allowed to visit me, if she arrived before 7 pm. It was 2:00 pm and Hélène had just gotten out of the shower. By 2:30 pm, Hélène was on the GO Train on her way downtown and by 3:30 pm, she was in the hallway outside my room. Because S.A.R.S. was still very much a part of our lives, Hélène had to don mask, gown, gloves, etc. before entering my room. She had asked the Social Worker not to tell me that she was on her way to see me, so when she appeared at my door, I was absolutely blown away! At first, I wasn't even sure who was there (because of the mask, gown, etc.). Hélène was able to stay with me until about 7:30 pm. She fed me my dinner and we had a wonderful visit until it was time for her to go. The next day, she was leaving for Montréal to visit her mother for Mother's Day, so I wouldn't be able to see her until Monday.

The next thing I knew, I was at Bridgepoint Health, which would become my "home away from home" for the next five and a half months. I was mostly in a semi-conscious state for the first few days and I would wake up periodically. It was like I had slept for three months or so. I had no idea how I'd gotten there and could not remember anything but soon was into a daily routine that involved a series of wonderful and interesting people that included nurses, doctors and personal service providers who were constantly buzzing over me with pills and needles, taking my blood pressure and generally just making sure I was OK.

Apparently, I was doing reasonably well, considering everything I had been through over the past three and a half months. Granted, I had lost a tremendous amount of weight (about 60 lbs.), but everyone told me I looked great and I know I was very anxious to resume my "normal" life! I seem to remember that I had a tendency to be somewhat depressed and I think I had more interest in sleeping than just about any other activity. I was certainly very happy to see Hélène every day and I was always telling her how much I appreciated the time she spent with me.

My physiotherapy progressed well and, during the next three weeks, I went from barely being able to sit up (with lots of support and assistance) to not only sitting on my own for 15 minutes or so but correcting my posture myself if I started to slouch or fall sideways and standing (with some assistance)! Hélène tells me it was wonderful to watch me get stronger and stronger every day. I experienced some muscle and joint pain but that was to be expected, considering I had spent 12 weeks in bed with very little therapy (due to my high blood pressure).

Slowly but surely, I learned to do things for myself and I was soon brushing my own teeth, washing my face, shaving (with an electric razor) and eating and drinking on my own. All Hélène had to do was supervise so I didn't shave my head by mistake (don't laugh, I came close a couple of times!) and of course to make sure I didn't choke. I'm told that my speech was easy to understand, although a little slower. But my vocabulary was excellent (no memory loss there, that's for sure) and I was apparently sounding more and more like the old Peter (so to speak!).

Towards the end of June, 2003, my regular Physiotherapist went on vacation for a week and was replaced by the head of the Physio department. Steve continued Alan's good work and was actually able to get me up and doing some new activities that I had never tried before.

Steve was gentle, encouraging and not afraid to try new things. He had me pushing a shopping cart (kind of a shuffle, actually) and one day, I walked up (and down) a small flight of three stairs! I was so excited that I was able to do this! I was rolling up and down the hall in my wheelchair when I got back to my floor yelling "Show me the stairs! Show me the stairs!" When I called Hélène to tell her, we cried together on the phone. My left leg still wasn't moving on its own and Steve had to assist me in moving it up to the next step, but the point is I was able to put all my weight on my left leg without pain or discomfort! This was such a major accomplishment, you have no idea! Two weeks before, we had been wondering whether I would ever walk again and now I was doing stairs! I suppose, in retrospect, this was an early indication of things to come. I will be eternally grateful to the whole Physiotherapy team, particularly Alan, Steve and Ljuba. Without their encouragement, I probably wouldn't have made the progress I did while I was in rehab at Bridgepoint Health.

In addition to physio, my daily routine included speech therapy with Ran and Kathleen and occupational therapy with Jennifer. All three of these wonderful, dedicated women are owed my appreciation and gratitude for helping me regain my independence and resume a relatively normal life.

Hélène was spending as much time with me as the hospital would allow. I was in so much discomfort, pain and fear, unable to walk, use my left arm and basically unable to take care of myself. I would fall asleep at night in tears when she couldn't be with me or when it was "lights out" and she had to go home, but I thank my lucky stars that the wonderful nurses and PSPs understood my plight so well. Hélène was such a help to me every day and would bring me my meal trays and eat each meal with me.

Speaking of mealtime, it was quite an adventure that I had to go through to develop a whole new process of eating. Ran, my speech therapist, was responsible for working with the dietitian to determine how well I could swallow. Initially, solid foods were simply not an option for me. I can't express enough how much I longed for a normal meal of steak and potatoes. I had been surviving solely on liquid food since my stroke several months before and I wanted French fries and a Big Mac so badly! At this point, I really wasn't sure that I was ever going to graduate at all from "Ensure", the standard hospital liquid food for such seriously afflicted patients. Man, did I ever celebrate when I began to realize that I was successfully chewing and swallowing scrumptious whole meals of meat and potatoes! You may find it difficult to agree with me on this, but those hospital meals were actually quite delicious. We always anxiously looked forward to the predetermined meal times and appreciated the various meals we were given every day. And, of course, I wanted to be able to eat "regular" food at our wedding reception!

Now to the bad news. Much to our dismay, S.A.R.S. had reared its ugly head again. Over the past few days, the rehab centre had gone from "simple" screening of all visitors (no temperature taken, just questions about visits to affected hospitals and whether visitors were experiencing aches and pains, etc.) to temperature taking (again!) and masks. As of 8 pm on May 29th, visitors were no longer allowed. The hospital chose to do this as a precaution, as it was the only health care facility in Toronto that had no cases of S.A.R.S. and they wanted to keep it that way. We certainly understood why they wanted to protect their patients, but it didn't make it any easier! Hélène and I were completely devastated. I depended on her so much to reassure me and to give me the personal touch that the nurses and nursing assistants didn't always have time to give. The whole thing was quite a shock. All we could hope was that it wouldn't take as long this time. The last restriction was seven weeks long, although Hélène was able to continue visiting me for the first three weeks because I was in the ICU. Things were very different this time. We had actually been told by staff at the hospital that the outbreak was far worse this time, so who knew how long it would take to get the "all clear"?

To look on the positive side of all of this, as Hélène told me, the first little while would actually be a blessing in disguise (for her, anyway) as it would allow her to catch up on all the things she hadn't had time for over the past three weeks -- opening the pool, getting an oil change, getting a haircut, sleeping (!!!), etc. Somehow, though, I knew the novelty would wear off really fast! We missed each other so much and I was feeling a little lost without her. All we could do was to be strong and look forward to the day we could hold each other again!

A couple of days after the "lock-out", Hélène purchased a pair of walkie-talkies and brought one of them to me at the hospital. She contacted the Social Worker on my floor, whose name was Ed, and asked him to meet her at the front door of the hospital that afternoon. She gave him the walkie-talkie, which he passed on to me. He then got me out of bed and into my wheelchair and pushed me over to the window of my room, where I could see Hélène standing outside and just below the window. She had the other walkie-talkie and we were able to talk to each other for several minutes. We actually did this several times over the next couple of weeks and I think it's what helped keep me sane. Hélène also brought me various Care packages, which she gave to Ed. He gave her my dirty laundry, which she washed and brought back the next time she came to "visit". One day, Hélène showed up with a collage of photographs of her and me, the boys, trips we had been on, Christmas and birthday celebrations, etc. on a piece of bristol board. Ed put the bristol board on my wall, in front of my bed, so that I could look at it whenever I was feeling particularly lonely (which was all the time!).

My roommate at the time was a very compassionate and friendly fellow by the name of Mario. He had been the victim of a car accident and had sustained considerable head trauma. He and I got along famously right from Day One and he "looked after" me during the entire period that Hélène couldn't be there. He was my saving grace! He was a real treat and a great source of entertainment. He had become my best friend and he and I would joke and laugh together, basically just allowing the time to go by without getting depressed.

Poor Mario was very unpredictable. One day, he was perfectly fine; the next day, he would be angry and almost violent. He was not taking to hospital life and routine all that well. He was a very personable and even humorous individual, but he could get angry if his medicine was not delivered and administered on time or in what he deemed to be the appropriate dosage. The poor man would scream at the nurses and PSPs on the floor whenever he thought he was not going to get the relief he so looked forward to throughout the day.

Mario was a considerate and lovable man, but he had no patience when it came to his "needs". I used to laugh at him and reassure him at the same time whenever he would "lose it". Mario was obviously not having a pleasant time, but he loved to joke and playfully flirt with the nurses. But then again, all the male patients seemed to be the same. Let's face it, spending countless hours in a hospital bed, day after day, uncertain of your fate or recovery prognosis, what else was one to do? I know that I was unsure of my future. I had come to believe that I probably wasn't going to get out of there.

During the S.A.R.S. "lockout" in particular, Mario and I would spend hours talking about our families, music and, most especially, what we would do when we got out of the hospital.

Mario had a brother and a sister who lived in the Toronto area and he was hoping to go and live with one of them, initially at least. His sister in particular was very attentive and would visit him regularly. We both found it difficult when no visitors were allowed, but at least we had each other! He even managed to talk me into going to Sunday Mass with him on a few occasions! Although I had never been a religious or spiritual person and probably never will be, I have to admit that, at the time, I enjoyed going and was able to find some solace in the peace and tranquility I found whenever I was in the chapel. I even thought that maybe going to Mass would make a difference and give me a chance at a renewed life.

I was wondering what was going to become of me and was thinking that, if I tried to talk to and get a little closer to God and let Him know I loved Him, appreciated Him and was willing to know Him and see Him a little better, that maybe He would be able to help me and fix the nightmare I was going through. Well, so far, nothing, and every once in a while, you hear of another tragedy or some pathetic loss of life or compromise to life and humanity and you wonder, who can be watching over us and keeping us safe? (Well, at least the good people, anyway.) Dad is a wonderful Christian. He always encouraged us to say grace before a meal and the family always got together for Christmas, Easter and Thanksgiving. He also always had us (the kids) attend Sunday School and then Church service when we were older. By the time I was 12, I was old enough to insist I didn't want to go, probably because, as a teenager, I just wanted to use the time to sleep in!

Well, as I said, I am not a churchgoer, but I have always respected other peoples' choices. Since my stroke, I can certainly comfortably say I love God. A couple of times, I believe I have said "How the heck can God do this to me? I have never been a bad person, I have never hurt anyone." I would never hurt anyone, I love animals and I am not racist, plus I always wish people the best.

On August 1st, 2003, Mario was discharged from hospital and, unfortunately, I lost touch with him. I just hope that, wherever he is and whatever he is doing, he is happy and healthy and I wish him all the best.

My second roommate at Bridgepoint was a delightful older gentleman by the name of Frank. He was quite a character and he also kept me entertained during the weeks we shared a room. Hélène and I had many laughs with him and thoroughly enjoyed his stories. He eventually moved on to a Nursing Home in the Peterborough area, I believe.

My last roommate was a young Oriental lad named Reno, who was married with a young child and another on the way. His mother, who spoke no English at all, was with him every day, taking care of all his needs much in the way Hélène did for me. His wife would come by after her work day had ended to relieve his mother and she would stay with him until visiting hours were over. He couldn't speak because of a breathing tube he had had inserted in his trachea, but certainly understood everything we said to him and would respond accordingly. When I was finally discharged on October 24th of that year, he cried when we said goodbye. Such relationships were special, emotional and sometimes very short-lived.

My D-Day (Discharge Day!) was a very emotional one for Hélène and me both, as well as for all the staff who had taken care of me all these months. Hélène brought in her camera and she took pictures of everyone, so that I would always remember them. I often look back on those pictures and find it difficult to believe how long it's been since I left there!

After my discharge, I was invited to come back to Bridgepoint to their "Stroke Clinic". Basically, every two or three months for a year or so, I would spend a couple of hours there, seeing the various therapists with whom I had worked when I was an inpatient. The idea was for all of them to track my progress after my release. I used to enjoy visiting everyone, seeing the nurses and PSPs, showing off how well I was doing. The staff always seemed really happy to see me and greeted me with loving, open arms. They were a wonderful group of caring people and I will never forget them and what they did for me.

CHAPTER 2:   WEDDING PLANNING

For most couples, the weeks and months leading up to their wedding day are fraught with tension, excitement and nervousness. Unless you've actually experienced this, it is difficult to describe the gamut of emotions that both the bride and groom-to-be will live through during this period. For Hélène and I, the time leading up to our wedding day was exciting, certainly; but more than that, in such a rather uncertain time in our lives, it gave us both something wonderful and positive to which we could look forward. One thing we were very certain of was (and is) our love for each other.

As I mentioned earlier, I had proposed to Hélène a week or so after my first stroke. While I had caught her somewhat by surprise, she accepted eagerly and we were both very excited. Unfortunately, fate then intervened and I had a second stroke and we were forced to put any talk of wedding plans on hold for the next two and a half months while I pursued my main objective of getting better. It wasn't until I had been transferred to Bridgepoint Health to begin my rehab that we set a date and planning began in earnest. After looking at a calendar, we decided on Saturday, September 27th, 2003 for our special day.

There are so many details to think of when planning a wedding and, fortunately for me, Hélène is a detail-oriented person. Once we had set the date, we obviously needed to find a location for the ceremony and the reception. Hélène searched the internet and found a web site that listed several potential venues in our area. After checking out prices and availability, we finally decided on the chapel at the Pickering Museum in Greenwood, not far from our home in Whitby. Hélène's son, Paul, had returned from Hawaii by this time and the two of them drove up to Greenwood to check out the location. In both their opinions, it was perfect! It was a quaint setting, not unlike a pioneer village, with many gardens and trees, very picturesque and, fortunately, it was totally wheelchair-accessible! I had told Hélène that, as long as she thought it would do the trick, she should book it then and there before someone else did, which is exactly what she did.

The next thing we had to deal with was the location for the reception. There was no question in our minds that our first choice was Krebs, the last restaurant we had been to before my stroke. The staff there had been so efficient and pleasant and the owners, Gary and Patricia, had been kind and welcoming, even though we had shown up there previously on Valentine's weekend without a reservation!

Hélène made a point of dropping in to the restaurant and asking the owners whether there was space available for our wedding reception. Fortunately, they were more than accommodating. In fact, we discovered a little while later that they don't normally cater to that type of event, as it ties up the staff and the tables on what is normally a very busy night for them (Saturday). Luckily for us, they thought we were a special couple and, after hearing about our situation, they agreed to make an exception. The pathway to a very special and momentous day was paved!

Obviously, you can't have a wedding without a minister and, again, fate intervened. Our neighbours across the street had recently been to a wedding and had been very impressed by the minister who had performed the ceremony. They managed to get his name and telephone number and Hélène contacted him immediately. He was available on the day we had selected and he and Hélène made arrangements for the three of us to meet at Bridgepoint. Over the next few weeks, we met with the minister, Peter, on three separate occasions as we shared our thoughts and feelings about marriage, relationships, commitment and love. We told him how we had met, what we each expected from this marriage and what type of ceremony we would like to have, including writing our own vows.

The next detail to deal with was the rings. Hélène had been scoping out the options in several of the local jewellery stores, but really hadn't seen anything that appealed to her. One day, while we were sitting and chatting at the hospital, it suddenly occurred to me that I used to play tennis in Newmarket with a wonderful Dutch gentleman who owns a jewellery store. The next day, Hélène gave him a call and arranged to go there to look at some of his pieces. Henning very kindly agreed to let Hélène borrow a few samples for a couple of days so she could bring them to me at the hospital and we could make our choices. This worked out very well, as we happened to like and selected the same rings! Hélène returned the samples to Henning the following day and placed the order for our respective wedding bands. Henning assured her they would be delivered in plenty of time for our wedding day.

Hélène went out for dinner one night with a close and very dear friend of hers, a lovely woman who had worked with Hélène a few years previous. Elise and I had met on a couple of occasions, but I really didn't know her all that well. Now I can safely say that she has become a special friend to both of us! Anyway, during the course of the dinner, Hélène asked Elise if she would be her Maid of Honor. Elise was thrilled; in fact she said it would be an honor! The two of them had great fun making plans and discussing some of the many details that are such a crucial part of putting together such a special day.

It proved to be just as easy for me to find my Best Man. This was obviously an important decision and one of many overwhelming details to take care of, because being hospital-bound, I had grown out of touch with most of my regular and best of friends. Doug and his wife, Jane, however, who I have known for over 30 years, had always stayed in touch and had been in to see me as often as possible. They had also been very attentive to Hélène, calling her regularly to see how things were going. I knew I could count on Doug to perform this important function and he agreed immediately, which gave me tremendous relief as such details were so emotional and important to me. Jane is the sister of one of my oldest friends, John, who I met shortly after moving to Renfrew. Anyway, I called Doug one day and asked him if he would be my Best Man and he said "Absolutely!" It was such a relief for me to know that this detail was looked after. As Doug lived relatively close by, he would look after getting me to the church on the big day.

Hélène asked her son, Paul, to give her away and we both asked Tyler and Corey to be Ushers. We then made arrangements with a local formal wear store for suits, etc. for all the men in the wedding party and Hélène and Elise proceeded to purchase their dresses, book their hair appointments, etc.

The principle details having been looked after, Hélène ordered the flowers for the church, a bouquet each for her and Elise, corsages for Hélène's mother and stepmother and boutonnieres for all the men. Of course, no wedding would be complete without music and Paul offered to play the recessional song on his guitar. As well, he and Hélène put together a c.d. compilation of appropriate background music, including the song that would be playing as they entered the church.

A close friend of ours, Carole (with whom Hélène had worked at the school board) offered to look after making up small organza bags filled with rose petals for each guest to throw after the ceremony, in lieu of confetti, which the museum had asked us not to use. Carole's fiancé, Daniel, graciously offered to be our official photographer and, for the reception, Hélène purchased disposable cameras for each table so Daniel would be able to enjoy himself without having to constantly go around the room taking pictures.

All in all, everything was falling into place very well. The icing on the cake was when the Program Director, Rehabilitation at Bridgepoint, who had become a dear friend and who, along with her husband, would be attending our wedding, offered the services of a PSP to accompany me on the big day. Arthur looked after getting me ready, showering me, shaving me and dressing me and was wonderfully attentive throughout the day. He even accompanied Hélène and me to our hotel after the reception, to make sure we got there safely and got settled in without incident.

As I had started coming home on weekends some time in July, for the wedding I was given an extra long pass to spend a few days with my loving wife. My mother-in-law had generously arranged for us to spend a few nights at a local hotel and some friends of ours from Indiana, who had flown into town just for the wedding, happened to be staying at the same hotel as us. Rich and Connie had only been married for about a year themselves and they graciously offered to take us out to dinner the night following our wedding. We had a wonderful time and had many laughs with them. They are a great couple who are, unfortunately, very, very busy and so, we haven't seen them at all since the wedding. We keep talking about going down to Terre Haute to see them, but somehow other things keep interfering! Hélène and I keep telling each other that we couldn't possibly work full-time in addition to all our current activities, as there isn't enough room in our busy schedule!

Hélène and I were so anxious for the big day! During the last ten days or so, Hélène made a countdown calendar for me which I kept at the foot of my hospital bed. Every day when she came in to visit me, she would change the number of remaining days so I could keep track.

One of the most important things we needed to do prior to the wedding was to purchase or lease a new vehicle to get me to the church and obviously for afterwards, when I returned home. The question was…what should we get?

I had had a couple of vans over the past several years which were handy for moving me, my wife and our boys to our various and sundry appointments and events. They were also practical for transporting my amp and guitar and my band mate's equipment whenever it was my turn to bring the band's musical instruments to gigs and practices.

This being the case, it was an easy choice. Just three days before the wedding, we took delivery of a brand new 2003 Chevrolet Venture van, this one equipped with a Turny seat, a seat that turns and swings outwards at the flick of a lever, then lowers on a chain driven belt via a remote control to move the seat in or out of the van as necessary, to the appropriate level so that I can seat myself easily. It then rises up and glides back into the van, at which point, the same lever unlocks the seat and allows me to turn myself into the van. As well, the van is equipped with a remote controlled lift that brings my 275 lb powered wheelchair in and out of the van so automatically that Hélène can easily do this herself within a few seconds. Hélène always says that if she had a quarter for every time she's been asked by passers by about the modifications we've had done to wheelchair-equip the van, she'd be a rich woman!

Hélène's mother came in from Montréal on the Wednesday prior to the wedding and she and Hélène came to Bridgepoint to see me on Thursday. It was the first time Magdeleine and I had seen each other since my stroke and she was pleasantly surprised at my progress. My own mother was hospitalized at the time and could not actually make the wedding herself but Dad and my sister and niece came down from Renfrew, as did five out of six of Dad's sisters, some from as far away as Edmonton. It promised to be a wonderful family reunion.

Before I knew it, it was Friday, September 26th. Hélène went home at her regular time and I stayed at the hospital so as not to see her on the morning of our wedding (tradition, don't ya know?). I still remember sleeping solidly that night, knowing that when I woke up, it would be our anxiously awaited wedding day.

CHAPTER 3: HERE COMES THE BRIDE

The morning of September 27th was initially somewhat disappointing as it was pouring buckets! Hélène reassured me that rain on your wedding day is supposed to be good luck, so I decided to just "go with the flow".

Hélène and her mother had made hair appointments for that morning and Elise, her 'Maid of Honour' was scheduled to meet them back at the house at about 1:00 pm. The wedding was scheduled for 5:00 pm. Paul and his friends, Ian and Rich, as well as Ian's girlfriend, Jordan, and Paul's girlfriend, Alex, also met back at our place and everyone got ready and drank a glass of champagne before leaving for the church.

Just as the ladies were putting the finishing touches on their makeup, Hélène happened to look out the window and, much to her delight, the sun was shining! It ended up being a beautiful hot and sunny afternoon and evening. It was a perfect afternoon for pictures outdoors and for gathering in front of the church before and after the ceremony. The setting at the museum was also superb!

Doug, his son Spencer, Arthur and I were finally ready to leave Bridgepoint at about 3:00 pm. We were a short distance away when Arthur realized he had forgotten the bag of medical supplies that the nurses had put together for me to use over the weekend (my meds, etc.), so he returned to the hospital and eventually met us at the church.

When we arrived at the church, most people were already there, with the exception of my bride. Although I had certainly participated in creating the list of invitees, my short-term memory deficit made it difficult for me to remember everyone who would be there. It was such a treat to actually see the faces of the people I love and to remember that they had been invited and had accepted. While people were entering the church, having been handed a program and escorted to their seat by one of the Ushers, there was soft classical music playing in the background. The flower arrangements were at the front of the church. Candles were lit throughout the church, the sun was shining through the stained glass windows and the birds were chirping in the trees. What a moment! I was so happy and so excited! I never stopped smiling till my eyes closed as my head hit the pillow that night.

After the initial greetings, complete with hugs and kisses from everyone, I waited patiently (alright, not so patiently!) for Hélène to arrive. After a few minutes, I was informed by one of the boys that she had arrived and was waiting outside in the car. It seems that my future father-in-law and his wife had gotten lost on the way to the church and, for obvious reasons, we couldn't really start without them! Finally, Paul saw them arrive and he and Alex met them outside. While Paul pinned the boutonniere on his grandfather's lapel, Alex pinned Isabella's corsage on her dress. We were now ready to start!

As Hélène and Paul approached the porch at the front of the church, Hélène noticed that there were rose petals not only on the porch but all the way up the aisle of the church. She quietly asked Paul what they were for and he told her they were for her! The stage was now set for a very special day!

As I obviously would be sitting in my wheelchair during the ceremony, an attractive antique wooden chair had been placed at the front of the church so Hélène could sit with me. Each of our chairs had a huge white bow on it and Hélène has told many people since then that, if the bow ever comes off my wheelchair, the honeymoon is over! So far, it is still in place and I, for one, have no intention of ever removing it.

Peter, our minister, had prepared some beautiful words based on what we had shared with him during our meetings. He talked about how we met, how much we had in common, how much we had been through together and what had brought us to this day. Hélène and I both cried while he spoke. When we exchanged our vows (prompted by Peter, so we wouldn't forget anything), we held hands and, again, cried tears of joy. We just kept smiling at each other – we both knew in our hearts that this was the best moment of our lives!

Once we had signed the registry, it was time to exit the church and Paul and Ian began playing the song Paul had chosen as our recessional, "Two Step" by the Dave Matthews Band. Somehow, the words seemed to Paul to be so appropriate and this was his way of contributing to the ceremony. Here are some of the words from the song, which you will see were perfect under the circumstances:

Hey my love do you believe that we might last a thousand years
Or more if not for this, our flesh and blood
It ties you and me right up
Tie me down

Celebrate we will, because life is short but sweet for certain
We're climbing two by two

To be sure these days continue
These things we cannot change

Paul and Ian did such a wonderful job! In fact, Paul was so intensely into the music that his fingers were bleeding by the end of the song! Afterwards, we all gathered outside on the front porch for hugs and kisses and many, many Kodak moments!

Tyler and Corey had decorated our van with a "Just Married" sign, as well as streamers and balloons and, once we got into it, we headed to Krebs for the reception where more surprises awaited us!

By the time my bride and I arrived at the restaurant, everyone else was already there. They all applauded when we made our entrance and I think the other patrons in the restaurant must have been wondering just what was going on!

The menu consisted of five or six choices, basically their banquet menu, and included a deliciously extensive salad bar, dessert and coffee or tea. In addition, Hélène's mother had generously donated the champagne for a toast prior to the meal. As Hélène and I had been living together for several years and really didn't need anything, we just asked our guests to cover the cost of their own meal and drinks, in lieu of wedding gifts. Everyone seemed very pleased with this suggestion, although there were a few people who decided to give us a wedding gift as well, which was much appreciated. As a special touch, we decided to make a donation to the Heart and Stroke Foundation on behalf of each of our guests.

Somehow, it seemed appropriate to support this particular association under these circumstances.

Paul and Ian had set up their instruments behind the "head" table and they entertained us all evening, which was a real treat. The members of my band, Tom and Wayne, also picked up the instruments and played a few tunes for us which added to everyone's enjoyment.

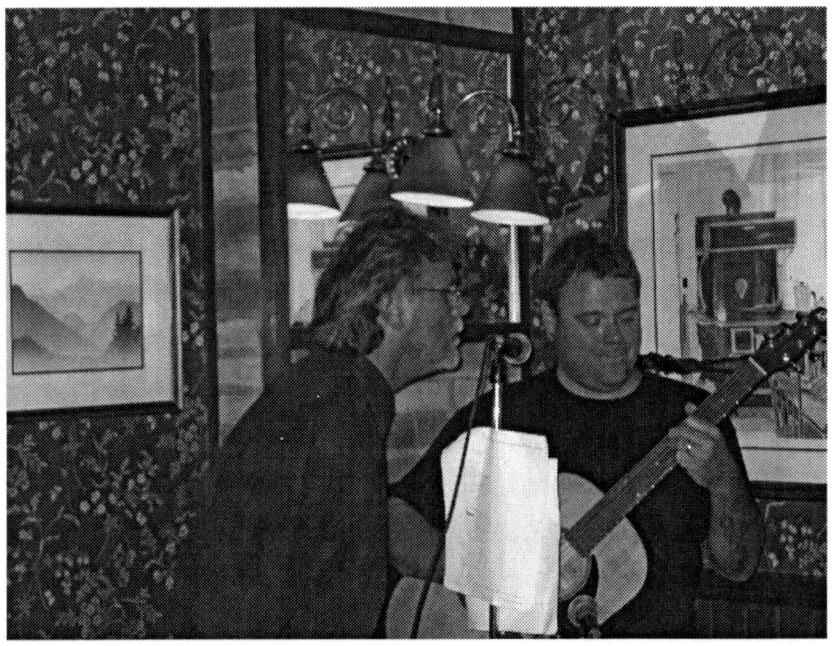

My former band mates, Tom and Wayne, performing at our wedding reception, September, 2003

Despite the fact that I had been hospitalized at this point for seven and a half months, I still managed to close the restaurant and leave for the hotel with my new wife at about 11:30 pm! I was extremely tired by the time we arrived in our room, but I was thrilled with the day and I looked forward to spending the next few days with my best friend!

CHAPTER 4: SPECIAL PEOPLE

The following are a few of the special people (professional and others) who touched my life during my hospital stay and since my discharge. I want them all to know how very special they are to me and how grateful I am to them for playing the crucial parts they did during my recovery efforts.

NURSES/PSPs, etc.	HOSPITAL
Kathy	Ajax-Pickering Hospital
Eva	Ajax-Pickering Hospital
Anna	Ajax-Pickering Hospital
Leslie	Ajax-Pickering Hospital Emergency Room
Ruth	Toronto Western Hospital 5A
Jen	Toronto Western Hospital 5A
Margaret	Mt. Sinai Hospital Intensive Care Unit
Kathi	Management, Bridgepoint Health
Ed	Social worker, Bridgepoint Health
Digna	Bridgepoint Health
Elizabeth	Bridgepoint Health
Georgina	Bridgepoint Health
Arthur	Bridgepoint Health
Patricia	Bridgepoint Health
Suzette	Bridgepoint Health
Chris	Social worker, Whitby Day Hospital

THERAPISTS	HOSPITAL
Alan	Bridgepoint Health (physio)
Ljuba	Bridgepoint Health (physio)
Jennifer	Bridgepoint Health (occupational)
Ran	Bridgepoint Health (speech and language)
Kathleen	Bridgepoint Health (speech-language pathologist)
Joanne	Ajax-Pickering Hospital (outpatient physio)
Thea	Ajax-Pickering Hospital (outpatient occupational)
Tim	Ajax-Pickering Hospital (outpatient speech and language)
Linda	Whitby Day Hospital (physiotherapy)
Janet	Whitby Day Hospital (physiotherapy)
Heather	Whitby Day Hospital (recreational therapy)
Agnes	Whitby Day Hospital (occupational therapy)
Sarah	Whitby Day Hospital (occupational therapy)

PHYSICIANS	HOSPITAL
Dr. Baker	Ajax-Pickering Hospital
Dr. Wang	Ajax-Pickering Hospital
Dr. Lozano	Toronto Western Hospital
The 4 Intensivists (specialists) at Mt. Sinai Hospital's Intensive Care Unit	
Dr. Tammy	Bridgepoint Health
Dr. Sommerville	Bridgepoint Health
Dr. Cook	Toronto Western Hospital
Dr. Guha	Toronto Western Hospital

ROOMMATES	HOSPITAL
Mario	Bridgepoint Health (my first roommate)
Frank	Bridgepoint Health (my second roommate)
Reno	Bridgepoint Health (my third roommate)
Ted	Toronto Western Hospital

I apologize for being so intent on the recognition kick here but these are people who, at one time or another during my recovery, I deemed responsible for enabling me to live again and overcome my new impairment. Thank you to all of you for being so instrumental in my recovery. You will forever be remembered and appreciated.

I apologize to anyone I may have forgotten and I am sure there may be some as I frequently have flashbacks and see you in front of me as part of a fond recollection of people who were very important and special to me.

While at Bridgepoint, after the initial period of adjustment, I became not only comfortable with the routine, but I was at home there. The staff was so friendly, helpful and encouraging and I even looked forward to the meals there. You could not complain about the food given at mealtimes and a snack was offered on a timely and much appreciated basis. Smiling and encouraging faces on the floor were the norm there and the doctors, nurses and social workers made regular appearances just to show their commitment, concern and support for all patients and staff.

A significant and vital part of my life and routine was that my wife was allowed to come in to see me every day and we enjoyed many hours together. This was so very special to us and I would cry whenever she was not able to be with me, either due to intermittent occasional hospital regulations or an appointment of Hélène's. Often, if a patient was away and therefore not able to eat their meal, the staff would give it to Hélène, so we frequently enjoyed meals like this together. We were so grateful for these opportunities.

My routine included an hour or two of physiotherapy, speech therapy and occupational therapy each day.

I have been home for more than two years now, having been discharged from Bridgepoint Health on October 24, 2003. I was quite accustomed to the routine there, lying in bed and then gradually awakening as each new day began, with the first few nurses and PSPs beginning their shifts usually at around 7:00 am, delivering and administering the various prescriptions, tending to full urinals, the occasional wet bed and basically getting the 50 or so patients on my floor comfortable and ready to start a new day. Given the excellent care we received at the hospital, we all actually looked forward to each new day.

At least we were alive and we could have confidence that we were being well cared for. Bridgepoint, 3 East was home to a number of us for weeks at a time and we usually had full and very interesting and dynamic days. I had no experience at all with hospitals before this tragedy, having had the good fortune to have been healthy all my life and, as I slowly became more cognizant of this strange, new routine and environment, I became quite secure and comfortable. Initially, I didn't understand what this stroke thing I had was all about and, as I learned more about my condition, I became more determined that I was going to lick this thing and simply get up and hoof it the hell out of here! As reality set in and time went by, I became aware that this was some serious shit I was into, and that recovery would not necessarily ever be complete. Whatever level of recovery I was to achieve, I knew it was going to be "A Long, Challenging Journey"! I was taught by the well-trained professionals there - the nurses, doctors and therapists - that any recovery was going to be long, hard and painful, with no guarantees. I had to accept that my own determination was going to have to play a key role in this new life. I am so grateful to the professionals at Bridgepoint Health for encouraging me and getting me to the point of being able to get in a vehicle again and go home with my wife, initially every weekend and eventually, to stay. It seemed to take forever to get home again and to assume a routine, albeit, somewhat modified with the wheelchair and lifts and such, but Hélène worked relentlessly and tirelessly coordinating contractors and various experts to get the necessary equipment and facilities in place and installed, in order to give me a reasonable chance at a new life.

CHAPTER 5: CHRONOLOGY OF MY REBIRTH

- I was reborn on Monday, February 17, 2003 – the day of my first stroke. On Friday, February 28, 2003 I had a second stroke.
- I proposed to Hélène on Monday, February 24, 2003 at 5:45 am.
- On Friday, May 9, 2003 I began a rehabilitation program at Bridgepoint Health. (I have no recollection at all of the period between February 17, 2003 and May 9, 2003.) I began to become aware of my life and my new condition at that time.
- On Saturday, September 27, 2003 Hélène and I were married.
- On Friday, October 24, 2003 I came home, finally discharged from rehabilitation at Bridgepoint Health.
- On Wednesday, October 29, 2003 I began outpatient rehabilitation at Ajax-Pickering Hospital.
- For Christmas, 2003 we were at home in Whitby with Hélène's Mom, Paul, Tyler and Corey.
- On Saturday, March 20, 2004 Hélène and I drove to Perth to pick up Cooper, our Golden Retriever puppy.
- On Saturday, March 27, 2004 Hélène threw me a 50+1 surprise birthday party.
- In May, 2004 we purchased and installed a pool heater which has allowed me to comfortably and regularly use the pool.

- In July, 2004 I began to play wheelchair tennis.
- On August 3, 2004 I was introduced to Taoist Tai Chi by Assunta Scaini.
- On Monday, September 13, 2004 I began taking Taoist Tai Chi Health Recovery classes at our local club in Whitby.
- On Friday, September 24, 2004 my Mom passed away peacefully in her sleep.
- On Sunday, December 19, 2004 we had Christmas dinner at home here with Dad, Brian and Linda, Diane, Megan, Tyler and Corey.
- For Christmas, 2004 we were in Montréal with Hélène's Mom, Dad and Stepmom.
- In June, 2005 I began to actually swim in our pool, working my way up to 15+ lengths every time I got in the water.
- In September, 2005 we began going to the Taoist Tai Chi Society's Health Recovery Centre and continue to go to its Health Recovery Week every month. The improvement to my overall mental and physical health as a result has been incredible.
- In late September, 2005 I began receiving acupuncture treatments on my leg, arm and hand.
- In early October, 2005 I was discharged from outpatient physiotherapy at Ajax-Pickering Hospital.
- On Saturday, December 17, 2005 we had another Frost family Christmas dinner here with Dad, Brian and Linda, Diane, Megan, Tyler and Corey.
- On Saturday, December 24, 2005 we had Christmas dinner at home here with Hélène's Mom, Paul, Tyler

- and Corey.
- For Christmas, 2005 we were home in Whitby with Hélène's Mom, Paul, Tyler and Corey.
- In February, 2006 we discovered another wonderful acupuncturist only five minutes from our home.
- On April 4, 2006 I began attending a new stroke-oriented therapy program at the Whitby Day Hospital.
- On Thursday, April 27, 2006 my Dad moved into a retirement home in Cobden, Ontario.
- On Tuesday, June 27, 2006 I was discharged from the rehab program at Whitby Day Hospital.
- On Friday, June 30, 2006 the sale of Dad's house was finalized and a wonderful chapter in our lives was closed.
- On Saturday, July 1, 2006 I swam in our pool without a life jacket for the first time.

CHAPTER 6:   A BUMP IN THE ROAD

On July 29 of last year, I experienced a bit of a setback. On that particular day, I was not feeling too well. I felt lethargic and my head was extremely thick and I had a hard time concentrating. I had a bit of a headache and my neck was very stiff and actually everything was tugging at me and I hurt or tingled all over. I was convinced there was something very bad going on inside my head. The pressure was intense and I insisted that I needed to go to the hospital. After taking my blood pressure, which had been elevated all day and was still 140/94, Hélène prepared me and we got in the van and drove to the Emergency department at Ajax-Pickering Hospital. It was just like days gone by, a déja-vu of sorts. After waiting three hours or so, they finally called my name and set me up in a bed in the observation area of the Emergency Room. My nurse, Leslie, took my vital signs and asked me several questions about how I was feeling and what had brought me to the hospital that day. She then told us that the doctor on duty would be coming in to see me shortly.

A short while later, Dr. Fashi came in and asked me more questions. She then indicated she wanted a CT scan done and they soon wheeled me over to Diagnostic Imaging. The results of the CT scan came in fairly quickly and Dr. Fashi came by and asked us when I had had my surgery, where it was done and who the neurosurgeon had been. She indicated there appeared to be some irregularity in the CT scan and, to be safe, she wanted to consult with a couple of other doctors and have the Internist on duty, Dr. Marcus, come in to talk to me.

The next thing we knew, I was being sent back to Diagnostic Imaging for chest x-rays. When we saw Leslie, we asked her what was going on and she indicated that the doctor had arranged for me to be transferred down to Toronto Western, to be seen by a neurologist. She also indicated that, despite having been on antibiotics off and on for more than five weeks, I still had a bladder infection!

Once we knew that the ambulance had been called to transfer me downtown, Hélène went home and picked up what I would need for my stay at Toronto Western, including my usual medication. She returned to Ajax-Pickering a short while later and the ambulance arrived around 10:30 pm.

I was taken by ambulance down the Don Valley by Paramedics Rob and Murray, who by the way are apparently much appreciated because the nurses indicated their respect for them. Isn't it nice to know that the appreciation of such important and professional people that have to work together is recognized and shared?

So, before I knew it, I was being whisked up the elevator of the Toronto Western Hospital and was laid in a hospital bed next to my new room-mate, Ted. Ted was an incredible man with the most amazing story. As I was attempting to position myself in what would hopefully be my temporary quarters, I had looked over and said hi to him, observing and subsequently realizing that he had obviously undergone a tragic experience. I noticed that he was not capable of using all of his limbs and that he was suffering from some type of paralysis, in some ways, similar to mine.

As we chatted and got to know each other, I learned that he had fallen at home and had broken two vertebrae in his neck. He had been a surveyor for York Region, obviously a professional in every respect and was quite disappointed to have been rendered incapable of going back to work. It became apparent that Ted was quite a family man with two wonderful stepdaughters, a charming, devoted wife and a new puppy. Did this remind me a little of someone else I knew? He's a very personable man, with an optimistic outlook on life. He told us that, whenever he starts to feel sorry for himself, he goes down to the floor where the children are who have never known life without a wheelchair and he realizes that he had 54 good years and is lucky to be alive. He has been at Toronto Western for about 10 weeks now and is waiting to be transferred to a rehab facility, where he hopes to be able to regain the use of his hands. Ted and I quickly became friends and promised each other to stay in touch.

This whole experience at the hospital this time was just like reliving my first stay two and a half years ago. Hélène and I had to wait for the resident, Dr. Cook, who was in surgery and wouldn't be up until 2:00 am. When he arrived, at 3:00 am, he showed Hélène my CT scan films and explained to her what he was concerned about.

Hélène and the doctor then came into my room, where I was dozing comfortably, woke me up and explained to me what the apparent problem was. There appeared to be evidence of hydrocephalus, which might be the cause of the pressure in my head. You'll remember that I had hydrocephalus or water on the brain when I first had my strokes. Anyway, Dr. Cook told Hélène to go home and get some rest. He said they would probably be doing an MRI but, as this was the beginning of the Civic Holiday weekend, nothing would be done until at least Tuesday. He did promise to try to rush things along a little, so that we wouldn't have to wait three days.

Hélène drove home, arriving at around 4:00 am. Although she was extremely tired, she was also somewhat pumped and couldn't sleep. She finally dozed off at about 5:30 am, only to be woken up by my telephone call at 9:00 am! Dr. Cook, who was a resident, had come in to see me with the neurologist. The neurologist asked me several questions about how I was feeling, what had brought me to the hospital, etc. He then informed me that they had now compared the previous night's CT scan to a film that had been done two years earlier when I was discharged from Toronto Western. Guess what? There was absolutely no change! Hence, no concern! He told me to go home and have a nice weekend! After all that worrying, there was nothing wrong with me that hadn't been there since the very beginning of my illness. I was so relieved!

At the same time, though, I couldn't help but wonder why I had been feeling so terrible the day before. For whatever reason, those feelings eventually went away and I never did find out what had caused them.

CHAPTER 7:   REHABILITATION

On March 10th of this year, while visiting my physiatrist for a further series of Botox injections, I told him that I wasn't too satisfied with the progress I had made thus far with my left arm. I indicated to him that I would have liked to pursue some form of therapy to continue to help improve the function of my hand and my arm. He told me about a short-term therapy program that might help and that it was located at the Whitby Day Hospital, just six minutes from our home! That alone is a godsend, considering our time is so precious and that we are always just so busy with our errands, my appointments and the endless chores we have. He said he would send over a referral and that we would hear from the folks there within the next couple of weeks.

Just a couple of days later, we received a phone call from the receptionist at Whitby Day Hospital, setting up an assessment time for me. I was to see them for two hours on Friday, March 24th.

At the appointed time, Hélène and I drove over there. I was seen by each of the members of the rehab team, including the physiotherapist, the recreational therapist, the occupational therapist, the social worker and the nurse. They each asked me a series of pertinent questions about my medical history, what therapy I had already done, my lifestyle, etc. and explained to me what their particular role would be in my rehabilitation, should I be accepted to the program. They told me a little about how they work as a team, for the most part specializing in treating people who have survived a stroke, as well as MS and other brain-injured, disabled patients. All in all, Hélène and I were extremely impressed right from the start and were hopeful that I would be accepted. They each had indicated that they would be meeting as a team at the end of that day and would make a decision about a program for me at that time. Someone would let me know what the outcome was within the next day or so.

Later that afternoon, I received a phone call confirming that I would be starting my rehab program at Whitby Day Hospital on Tuesday, April 4th. I would be attending twice a week, for 12 weeks and would be there from 11:00 am to 2:00 pm. What a relief! Hélène and I were so pleased and excited to find out I had been accepted. This would be a new chapter in my rehabilitation story. I tell you, it was like my life had started over. I was so ecstatic and enthused that such a program even existed, let alone that it was so accessible and convenient to our home.

Over the next 12 weeks, I worked with this amazing team of professionals in pursuit of the highest level of recovery I could possibly achieve. Each day, my session would start with physiotherapy where I would work with Linda and Janet on stretching and bending my legs and walking with my side walker and on the parallel bars. They would correct my posture while sitting and encourage me to give my right arm and hand "a vacation" by using my left side more.

After lunch, we would usually play cards or do some other mentally stimulating activity with Heather, our recreational therapist.

Occupational therapy involved working mostly on my left arm and hand with my two therapists, Sarah and Agnes. These two women (and all the others) are so knowledgeable! They impressed me so much with their concern, care and dedication.

I also had occasion to meet with Chris, the social worker on the team, to get some suggestions from him on ways to relieve stress and relax a little more. He loaned me some tapes and exercises on relaxation to take home, which I found very helpful.

I met with Lynn, the team nurse, on two or three occasions as her participation in my therapy was on an as needed basis. She frequently monitored my blood pressure and kept track of my weight with the aid of a huge portable scale that was available at the hospital and with which people in wheelchairs could be weighed. In fact, she weighed me in my wheelchair the other day and she determined my weight to be a trim-and-slim 185 lbs or 84.6 kgs. Hélène and I were pleased. I weighed 220 lbs when I had my stroke and dropped to as low as 160 lbs during the seven and a half months I spent in hospital during my rehab and recovery, enduring G-tube fed liquid meals. Now, after completing a series of physiotherapy sessions and getting my appetite and eating ability back to normal, I am enjoying delicious and healthy meals daily.

I felt very much that everyone really cared for me, something we all need once in a while.

In retrospect, having now been discharged from the program, I can say that although I have certainly improved in many areas (in fact, my assessment score doubled over my score upon my initial admission), I could certainly benefit from further therapy. I understand that continued participation in this program is an issue of provincial funding - an example of where our Health Care system falls seriously short. I am a stroke survivor still far from totally recovered but I certainly could still improve; yet my therapy program, for the time being, has ended.

SECTION SIX – RECONSTRUCTION (THE PEOPLE IN MY LIFE)

CHAPTER 1: PEOPLE IN YOUR LIFE

People come into your life for a Reason, a Season or a Lifetime.

Reason:

When someone is in your life for a **Reason,** it is usually to meet a need you have expressed outwardly or inwardly. They have come to assist you through a difficulty, provide you with guidance and support, to aid you physically, emotionally, or spiritually. They may seem like a godsend, and they are.

They are there for the **Reason** you need them to be. Then, without any wrongdoing on your part or at an inconvenient time, this person will say or do something to bring the relationship to an end. Sometimes they leave you through death. Sometimes they walk away. Sometimes they act up or out and force you to take a stand. What we must realize is that our need has been met, our desire fulfilled, their work is done. The prayer you sent up has been answered and it is now time to move on.

Season:

When people come into your life for a **Season**, it is because your turn has come to share, grow, or learn. They may bring you an experience of peace, or make you laugh. They may teach you something you have never done. They usually give you an unbelievable amount of joy. Believe it! It is real! But they are with you only for a **Season**.

Lifetime:

Lifetime relationships teach you **lifetime** lessons, those things you must build upon in order to have a solid emotional foundation. Your job is to accept the lesson, love the person/people (any way) and put what you have learned to use in all other relationships and areas of your life.

Be who you are and say what you feel because those who mind don't matter and those who matter don't mind.
                                        Dr. Seuss

It is said that love is blind but friendship is clairvoyant.
                                        Anonymous

CHAPTER 2: ROUTINES

For almost anyone, routines provide a level of comfort that allow a person to feel secure, creates a certain degree of expectation and minimizes surprises. I don't know about you, but I have never liked surprises. Even before I got sick, I did not appreciate anything occurring that I was not fully prepared for or expecting. I suppose it had something to do with my perfectionist, type "A" personality. I always preferred to be prepared to respond to or solve the various situations I came up against whenever and as they arose, whether work-related or even a social situation such as planning a trip or a project or job around the house. I just hated surprises or anything that might interfere with efficiency or progress. To tell you the truth, I think I could and did handle any surprise quite well, particularly before I got sick. But now, since many of my facets are compromised, I certainly don't need surprises, nor can I afford any such deviations from the norm and I hate it when something happens for which I wasn't prepared.

One of the "calms" that occurs every day that I have now become accustomed to is an important and regular part of my daily routine. This includes the daily visit of any one of the many homecare workers assigned to me. Every day, one of these people comes to give me either a shower or what is called "peri-care". Showers are a particularly delicate process when the patient is paralyzed and literally has no function on one entire side. A significant part of my nightmare, of course, is the paralysis that I now have on the entire left side of my body including my left hand and leg, which leaves me unable to walk or play guitar any more. I am unable to shower or bathe myself now, so we have PSWs (Personal Support Workers) come in seven days a week to help me groom and dress for my day.

These individuals are very special people. They seem to understand a patient's needs and vulnerabilities. In my case however, I am pretty resilient and over the time I have been undergoing my rehab, I have become quite capable of balancing and hobbling on my one good foot. I can stand as the PSW pulls my boxers down and positions me to get to my shower bench and prepares to give me my shower. I have become quite capable of maintaining my balance and, in most cases, I can direct most of my personal care. Remember, I have had a quite serious brain surgery and I am often very uncomfortable in my head and can't always remember all the intricacies of things as seemingly simple as the usual daily routine. Even so, I have learned to systematically reassemble many of my needs and routines.

Let me tell you about these amazing helpers: Tom, Leanne, Susan and Debbie are my regular weekday attendants. They are the absolute best, so knowledgeable and naturally talented, they come in Monday to Friday to bathe me and help me get dressed. Susan and Debbie take me through a wonderful series of range-of-motion exercises for my left arm and leg that make me feel so wonderful and which I appreciate so much. The stretching of my limbs brings such relief considering the tightness and tone that is so uncomfortable down my left side. They are always punctual and so considerate and are the best when it comes to caring for their clients and the top-notch job they do.

Tom is the kind of person that anyone afflicted as I am would want and hope to have assigned to his/her care. Tom is a special kind of person. He understands the needs of those in his care, plus he has an amazing sensitivity and an incredible sense of humour, always entertaining me with his jokes and his unending repertoire of songs and jingles. He helps me to shave, which I have become able to do by myself for the most part. He helps me get dressed in whatever I have decided to wear that day. He also makes our bed and straightens and tidies the bedroom for us. Tom is extremely professional and understands what his clients need and are going through. This is very important to any patients who may be struggling with the day-to-day realities of their issues and medical problems. For a stroke victim, for example, the PSW needs to have a thorough understanding of the patient's physical difficulties and limitations in order to assure his or her safety and well-being. Caring for a stroke patient even requires a reasonable understanding of his or her medical status because, quite often, there could be depression or nervousness that should be handled very carefully. Tom has no difficulty understanding or dealing with any of these complicated details. I am lucky and fortunate that I seem to be aggressively attempting to avoid and overcome any of these weaknesses.

Tom's employer, St. Elizabeth Health Care, should be proud of the job they have done in providing the level of service they have and they should be pleased to have a dedicated employee like Tom.

Another special person in the extended series of people who provide such excellent homecare is Susan. As a registered nurse, she also has a thorough understanding of her clients' care requirements and is able to calmly, quickly and efficiently provide the necessary services to her clients. She is extremely knowledgeable and is very dependable and reliable. You can set your watch by her and Tom's arrival times. They are truly professionals. In addition to providing the same routine homecare as Tom, Susan also puts me through an extensive series of range-of-motion exercises, which always make me feel so much more vibrant and relaxed.

Leanne is one of the most recent additions to my care program. She actually initially started coming to the house on weekends only and then began coming in during the week for a short period when Tom was absent. As Tom's schedule has recently changed, Leanne is now coming in on Wednesday and Friday every week. Leanne is a bright, chipper, friendly and warm person. She has two young children and comes in with an endless array of humourous and informative "what the girls did yesterday!" type of stories. She is very entertaining, as well as warm and caring. I truly enjoy having her here and feel very safe and adequately cared for in her competent hands. She has a very accurate and realistic perspective on life, care and what a patient's actual requirements are. She has a compassion that is sometimes lacking or hard to find in this type of service.

The weekends are covered by Tom, Leanne, Nicole, Paul or one of a handful of other PSWs from St. Elizabeth Health Care who work the occasional weekend within the month. As a general rule, the same people seem to return or are usually rotated in every month, which makes accepting the process so much easier and bearable for the client since they already know the routine. Having and getting new and different people often and without notice is so annoying and makes things in a stricken client's and his partner's life very frustrating.

Patricia was a recent addition to the service complement who was coming in on Wednesday afternoons for three hours until, unfortunately, recently leaving the company. She made my lunch, did laundry, put me through my vital and so important "range of motion" exercises and generally helped Hélène and I out wherever she could. We were truly lucky to have her! I miss her valuable therapeutic care.

Debbie is a recent refreshing, professional and extremely knowledgeable addition to the complement of homecare service providers. Actually, I have found a particular area of her expertise to be the "range of motion" exercises. She understands my physical shortcomings and helps me with appropriate exercises so well. Thank you, Deb. I appreciate your work so much.

This certainly is a specialized little world where appreciation, dignity and respect surely are the key to one's comfort and happiness and actually contribute to a patient's outright survival. I truly and sincerely need and want to take this opportunity to recognize and personally congratulate these terrific people. Thank you! Thank you! Thank you!

CHAPTER 3:   TWO SPECIAL ANGELS

There are so many terrific people who are looking after my best interests. Let me tell you about a couple of other special people who have touched my life.

Angie is my wonderful personal trainer, who comes in to work with me once a week during the school year. As her "real" job is as an Educational Assistant at a local elementary school, she can only fit one visit in per week between September and June. During the summer months however, she is off during the day and we usually manage to schedule her in twice a week.

Angie works with me on a series of exercises, including 'range of motion' and other stretching and mobility movements with my arm and fingers and my leg and foot. It always feels so good. I am getting some voluntary movement back in my fingers and hip, but I cannot bend my arm, elbow or knee voluntarily as yet. I am hopeful, but only time will tell.

During the summer months, Angie and I try to go in the pool at least once every week, working on swimming, stretching, walking, etc. It was actually during one of these sessions last summer that I discovered that I could do a scissor kick while swimming across our pool! Depending on the weather, Angie and I will either go to the driving range to hit a bucket of golf balls during our second weekly session, or simply work on my 'range of motion' exercises indoors.

Angie has recently put me on to a co-worker of hers who also teaches at one of the local community colleges. Angie told him about me and my physical condition and he has recommended that I try paraffin wax treatments to loosen up my left hand. When I mentioned this to my physiotherapist at the Whitby Day Hospital, she was hesitant at the idea because of her concern for the hot temperature of the wax. I'll certainly check it out and we'll have to see whether this treatment makes sense in my situation. As I've said before, I'm willing to try anything out. What have I got to lose?

When I was a patient at Bridgepoint Health, I was being given wonderful full-body massages once a week from a young gentleman by the name of Gavin, who lived nearby in the Beaches area of Toronto with his then fiancée, Donna. Gavin would come to the hospital for an hour each week and he always succeeded in making me feel so much better, especially considering the fact that I was bed-ridden for the most part other than when I was at my various therapy sessions.

Then, when I was discharged from Bridgepoint, Gavin offered to drive to our home to continue my weekly massage sessions. Needless to say, I took him up on his offer! He would concentrate on specific areas of my body, depending on where my aches and pains happened to be that week and I truly appreciated his amazing talent. I felt so relaxed afterwards!

Gavin continued to come out to our home on a weekly basis for about two years. He always had wonderful stories to tell me about his young family. He and Donna had married by then and had a beautiful young son named Nicholas. In fact, they invited Hélène and me to their wedding and we had a wonderful time. During my massages, Gavin and I would talk about CSI – one of our mutually favorite television shows and compare notes on that week's episode. We always had a few laughs and enjoyed each other's company.

With all the different activities in which I became involved during that period, including Tai Chi, physiotherapy, my personal trainer, etc. I eventually realized that it was becoming increasingly difficult to schedule Gavin in on a regular basis and I reluctantly had to cancel his services. Who knows? Maybe someday I'll give him a call and see if we can start up again. I sure appreciated his work!

CHAPTER 4: SPECIAL WORDS ABOUT AND FOR CAREGIVERS

Caregivers are a stroke survivor's "lifeline to the world." They are also the nearest "target" when he/she is feeling angry or frustrated at what has happened to him/her and the stroke survivor will simply easily and quickly lash out at them. There is just no one else handier. Caregivers MUST also make arrangements to have "time out" for themselves. Also, it is imperative to educate immediate family and friends about these needs. It is also very important to try to be specific. Failure to do so may result in serious misperceptions.

The caregiver is the one facing the obstacles when their "loved one" or "stricken subject" has had something as serious as a stroke. Quite often, friends and family members just seem to become scarce when confronted with the new special needs.

The stroke survivor is still the same person "inside" but their life is just never quite the same anymore. The most "beloved" name in our vocabulary is spelled **c-a-r-e-g-i-v-e-r**. We can never thank or appreciate them enough.

CHAPTER 5: IT'S ONLY LOVE

As I mentioned earlier, Hélène and I have three terrific sons between us. Son #1 (Paul) is a young adult who turned 25 at the end of last summer. He seems to have his shit together, as they say. Paul's our globe-trotting, musically talented son who is currently living in Toronto, working at the Air Canada Centre. About a year ago, he and his girlfriend decided to move back here from Vancouver, in order for her to complete her schooling to become a teacher. They knew even before coming here that they would be heading back to B.C. as soon as possible and that Colleen would work while Paul attends school. Well, he applied to a college in Nelson, B.C., taking music (his passion) and looking forward to taking in all that can be enjoyed from anywhere on the West Coast. At this time (July, 2006), they have moved to Nelson and have secured jobs at a local hotel – Paul as a Bar Supervisor and Colleen at the front desk. They found a beautiful home on the side of the mountain in the village and are sharing it with another couple, good friends of theirs.

Paul is a personable individual with a sunny disposition. He is a deep thinker, a philosopher of sorts. He is very much into the Dalai Lama, Deepak Chopra and anything natural or spiritual. He's a vegetarian, a nature lover and a serious conservationist. Paul knows his course in life.

Paul and his mom are very close. In fact, he walked her down the aisle to give her away at our wedding a couple of years ago.

For your reading pleasure, you will find the poem Paul has written for my book at the end of this chapter. Enjoy!

Son #2 (Tyler) is also a young adult who turned 20 last summer. Tyler is in the process of discovering himself and establishing his future direction. He is a bright boy, a pleasure to have around and has an amazing artistic talent. He is considering taking an art program at University, so I'm sure we'll be able to view his talent in a gallery in the future.

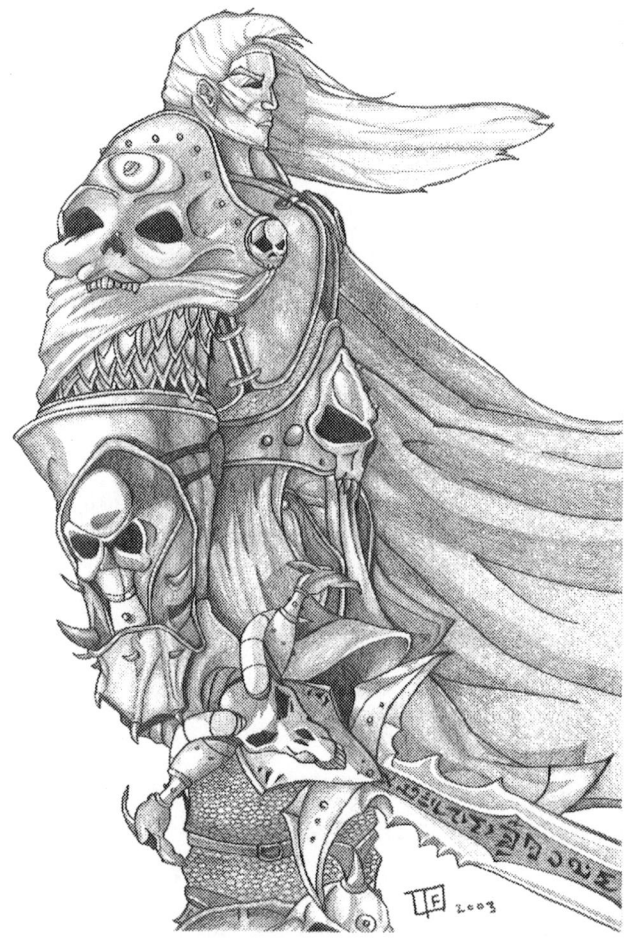

Another of Tyler's creations

Son #3 is blowing us away with his academic prowess. Now at the end of his grade 10 year, Corey seems to effortlessly pull off 80s, is popular with his friends and his teachers, and is also taking drum lessons and can often be heard beating away at his drum kit in the music room downstairs. At the end of last June, he wrote his grade 9 finals and "aced" his tests. We can only hope for more of the same this year! I just threw him a toonie to buy himself a treat for his walk home after school today. I folded a $5.00 bill into his palm yesterday and told him it was for doing nothing but to keep it up and wished him good luck with the rest of the school year and to double check his work. Gad, it seems like yesterday, we were going through the same thing ourselves. Well, his grade 10 year has been nothing but awesome and we have just received his final report card. As usual, Corey has made us proud!

An incredible part of the boys' taste in music is that it appears to be a little more sophisticated than mine ever was. For whatever reason, they seem to enjoy the exact same music that my wife and I used to like – Led Zeppelin, the Beatles, Black Sabbath, Nirvana, etc. I find this tremendously uncanny, but it makes me terribly proud at the same time. Of course, the years and technology have played their role in music. If the boys need a certain tune, they download it to either save it to CD or save it on their IPods or MP3 players. There is no shortage of music in our household. We are just amazed that the popular music most listened to in our home is the same stuff we were and still are listening to. Our chats at the breakfast and dinner table are about the same artists and we appreciate the same souvenir t-shirts and occasionally find them swapped for the day. Thank goodness, we seem to be bypassing the rap and the raunchier stuff.

It seems as though Paul has become an amazing musician overnight as he is starting to play single gigs. We are so proud of all our boys. Mom played piano all her life and she passed her piano on to my niece, Megan, who also seems to enjoy playing. Tyler and Paul both play guitar and, as I mentioned earlier, Corey plays drums. All three of these boys are so cool and capable and thoughtful with their young lives ahead of them.

Also in our lives there is my loving mother-in-law, Magdeleine, my father-in-law, Louis and my stepmother-in-law, Isabella, who are all so caring, intelligent and supportive. They provide us with an interesting and healthy perspective. I also am very fortunate to have the most wonderful wife a person could ever ask for. Despite my current situation, I am very much loved and appreciated.

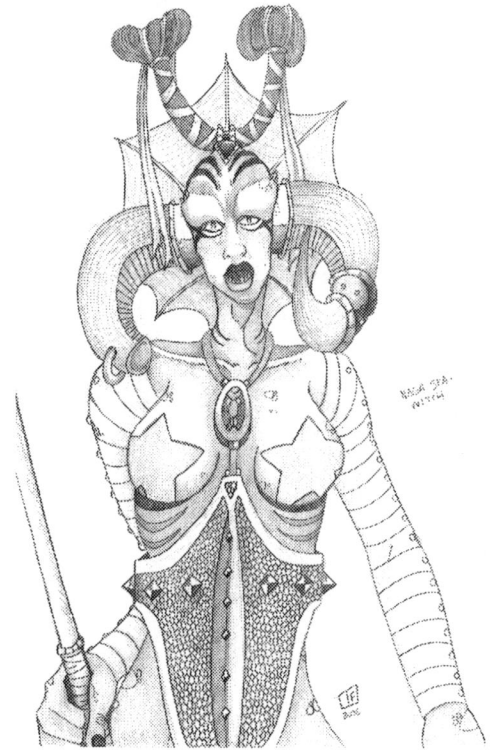

Another product of Tyler's imagination

Peter Frost

In Loving Hands

"You have to stop worrying."
That's what the Dr. said.
As alarm clocks keep ringing;
Now I can't get out of bed.
Maybe this time it's gone too far.
What time could it be?
This job's not a life, home in my car,
Yesterday I was doing fine.
I'm not done with this living.
Work myself to the bone.
Always getting and giving.
Time won't keep me down for long.
Headlines starting to slow down;
While the faster my heart races.
Pictures getting blurry around me;
Reaching out as my thoughts erase.
This is the big one.
Proudly reaching for the light.
When I awake sometime next year,
Please try not to cry.
Now I beg and I pray,
Buried under the desire to walk.
Did I take too much for granted?
Mostly tied myself up in knots?
I know that true progress
Is something we can all attain.
Things might even get better,
Without ever being the same.

Time makes us grow so fast,
The stages always come and go.
Just trying to plan for the chance,
To love my life and take it slow.
Life shouldn't be what scares you.
If you trust in a master plan.
It may put you in the hardest spot,
But leave you in loving hands.

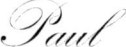

CHAPTER 6: NEIGHBOURS FROM HEAVEN

Hélène and I and our boys are blessed with our wonderful neighbours. Ever since we moved into our current neighbourhood, we have experienced the best friendships and neighbours a homeowner could ever hope to have. When we bought our current house, which is the cutest 1,600 square foot back-split, we painted all the bedrooms and made it our home. It is quite common that moving into a new home means that you adopt the previous owner's décor. This home was certainly cute but a few of the rooms just had to be repainted in the appropriate colours of our family's choosing.

We had picked a moving-in day in late August that enabled us to get right down to painting all the bedrooms and that is what we did, two days before the moving van arrived. We painted all three bedrooms but we didn't have to touch the family room downstairs, the kitchen or the living/dining rooms. The kitchen was a tastefully and immaculately decorated brand new Home Depot kitchen which I believe was actually what sold us on the house.

While taking a break from painting, we were pleasantly surprised by a group of people who suddenly appeared on our front lawn. They were some of the nice people who happened to be our new neighbours who had simply come over to welcome us to the neighbourhood. They introduced themselves (there were about 12 of them) and they immediately began telling us how happy they knew we were going to be with our investment. Next, one of them gave us a computer-printed list of all of their names, addresses, home phone numbers and children's names, which immediately made us feel comfortable and told us that we had picked a good neighbourhood. We smiled to ourselves as we took in the neighbourly introductions.

As it turned out, we were absolutely right in our initial impression of the nature of these wonderful neighbours. When I got sick and was hospitalized and Hélène's life was thrown into a tailspin, the neighbours all rallied around her and the boys and did everything they could to help out. They helped with chores and small (and some not so small!) jobs around the house, they ran errands, a few of them even drove the kids to and from their various commitments, drove Hélène to and from the GO train station when she came to visit me and even invited her to share meals or have a drink with them on more than one occasion!

Since I've been back at home, they have continued to be supportive and kind to both of us. We have never regretted our move into this wonderful neighbourhood. Even our newest neighbours, who moved in since I was discharged from hospital, have blended in nicely and also found ways to help us out and have become close friends of ours. We consider ourselves extremely fortunate to have found Dave and Heather, Dave and Theresa, Maralynne and Karen, Dale and Bonnie, Mark and Karen (and Luke, too!), Therese and Peggy, Roger and Jean, Marie and Des, Laurie, Kathy, John and Tracy, etc., etc. Then of course there's Adrian and Nancy and Steve and Jennifer, who live up the street and around the corner from us. Thanks, guys! You are truly neighbours from heaven!

Life can be good when you have good friends, good neighbours and also, when you earn, deserve and receive such good support and good customer service. We have a great network of friends that appears to be growing all the time. You just can't take such relationships for granted. Peoples' lives are busy and, quite often, you will encounter many people who are just too busy and who don't seem to have the time of day for you, even though you might expect differently of them. Fortunately, we have not encountered this situation in this neighbourhood. It always pays to be friendly and to always take the time to say "Good morning, how are you?" or "Good day!" Not only is it a sign of respect but it is an indication of appreciation and just simple, basic courtesy.

I have wanted to mention this about our unique neighbourhood. Never before, have I encountered such caring and well wishing people than what we have in this neighbourhood. These people, our dear friends, are truly wonderful. They have figured out what they want in life, what's good for their children and families and what they want as part of their day to day lives. These folks are constantly contributing to maintaining or increasing their property value and show all their immediate neighbours on a daily basis how much they appreciate and respect each other. These are the absolute fundamentals in creating and maintaining a balanced life, valued friendships and good cooperation.

We are very lucky to have found this home and this neighbourhood. The neighbours are second to none. Just imagine: someone in the neighbourhood goes away on a cruise for a week; then, a few days later, one of the neighbours notices no activity at the vacant house. The natural inclination then simply becomes to speak to a few of the other neighbours, to attempt to learn the nature and duration of the absence and explain the lack of activity and any of them go ahead, investigate and confirm that all is okay with that neighbour's house. The usual pattern is that someone will go over, knock on the door, check that all windows are intact and locked, look in and walk around the house and determine that all is clear and let a couple of other immediate neighbours know of the outcome of the inspection. It has even been common place that calls are made to the vacationers' family members to confirm that all is okay. This neighbourhood is known for treating each other as family and instills a solid "peace of mind". It truly is a gratifying and comfortable feeling and certainly contributes to the overall value, comfort and security within the neighbourhood.

There are numerous ongoing examples of wonderful, caring and compassionate people in this neighbourhood. I can't help but point out how Dave F. has been a constant and solid rock to everyone in the neighbourhood, whether it has been to solve a simple electrical problem or repair a faulty faucet, he has always been there with his limitless inventory of tools, experience, expertise and laughs to save the day. Not to mention the numerous times he has helped a few of us with our pool heater pilot lights. Dave is always there with his natural professionalism and great sense of humour. It just so happens this is the only way he knows how to work. He always responds with his famous "No problem! Give me a shout if you have any more problems." Dave F. and Dave W. have also been known to magically show up, unsolicited, for a few of us on those really challenging winter days with their snow blowers, bless their hearts.

CHAPTER 7: THE GFCI FROM HELL

Shortly after moving into our new home in August, 2002, we got involved with the inherent characteristics of the house and started to become more familiar with the neighbourhood and, of course, some of the neighbours. Aside from painting, touching up and repairing some of the wooden mouldings, I got down to replacing some of the electrical receptacles and switches and, of course, the appropriate wall plates. At some point, while replacing the plugs and switches in the master bedroom, I allowed my screwdriver to touch the contacts, arcing and causing a simple, quick short-circuit, resulting in all the power to the light switches and plugs in the room going out. As I was reasonably experienced in household electrical work, I understood the seemingly simple problem and went downstairs to the breaker panel to switch the lights back on. I was unsuccessful however, as I determined that there was apparently some kind of a strange, unconventional arrangement with the wiring in the master bedroom.

To be specific, even though I was able to determine that all of the switches in the breaker panel were in the proper position, I could not get the lights or any of the various fixtures in our bedroom to come back on. The damned TV, VCR, DVD player and digital cable box weren't coming on. Also, strangely enough, I couldn't get the ceiling light or ceiling fan to work. Well, this just didn't make sense.

So we called our magic man, Dave, our resident "across the street" master electrician and asked him what he thought the problem might be. I was actually thinking that I was going to have to go right inside the walls and run some new wiring to bypass the problem; however, fortunately, Dave was able to offer up the solution which was incredibly astute on his part and for which I, once more, will be eternally grateful. Dave indicated that he thought he recalled that the previous owner had intercepted and cut in to the bedroom circuit when he replaced a regular casement window with a patio door and actually even recalled that he had installed a GFCI on the outside wall to serve a receptacle for the pool pump. We had also recently installed a new patio lamp set and so, we were slowly adding to the overall load on the circuit. Dave pointed out that it didn't seem appropriate to have a GFCI in such a configuration and offered to come back later to correct our situation. Dave discovered that the GFCI was wired in such a manner that it was actually protecting the entire bedroom circuit. He skillfully corrected the problem by branching it off the circuit instead of directly feeding and protecting the circuit. A couple of moments later, he (with his 14 year old son Danny assisting) had everything running smoothly and shining brightly. The GFCI from hell was no more!

CHAPTER 8: ALL TOGETHER NOW

My Best Man, Doug and his wife, Jane, had been very close friends of Hélène and I since we lived together in Holland Landing, the four of us enjoying a few dinners and many bottles of wine.

One day, during the spring following my discharge from rehab, Hélène and I were sitting in Doug and Jane's kitchen, chewing the fat so to speak. We ended up discussing Corey's interest in pursuing drum lessons and one day hopefully starting a band with his buddies. Doug and Jane's son, Spencer, had already been playing drums for some time and had a drum kit of his own set up in his room. As our house is a backsplit, sound was an obvious factor in our case. Doug suggested the possibility of sound-proofing a room where Corey could set up his kit and pound away without disturbing the rest of the household. What a plan! As it turns out, my office, which was in the basement, was no longer being used as an office and would be the perfect spot for a music room.

During the course of our conversation, Doug generously offered to help us out by undertaking the renovations for us. He had experience in this sort of work, having previously built a beautiful finished apartment for his Mom in the basement of their 2,800 sq. ft. home.

Doug first prepared to sound-proof and finish the ceiling and boxed over the heating ducts. A major part of completing the room was to drywall and "mud" the walls and corners. Before long, the room was taking shape. It was getting close to "move in" condition. Once Doug had finished his part of the job, we purchased what we thought would be suitable paint and asked our son, Paul if he would do the honours. In no time at all, the room was done but, somehow, it didn't seem to look quite right. The colour we had chosen was somewhat "washed out" for a musician's lair! As Paul was heading out of town the next day, we asked our handyman, Adrian, his opinion about the colour. (As I am colour-blind, I was certainly not in a position to express an opinion one way or the other.) Adrian agreed that the colour wasn't quite vibrant enough for a 15 year old musician and he and Hélène discussed at length what a suitable colour would be. As Corey's drum kit is red and would be set up in front of the back wall of the room, we decided to go with red on that wall and a very pale blue on the other walls, with the accents (ceiling box, window frames, baseboards, light switch covers) in bright blue. Adrian did the job while Hélène and I were at Health Recovery Week and, when we came back, it was all done. What a beautiful room it turned out to be. In the next few days, Corey set up his drums again and put up a fine collection of rock music posters, including a shrine themed around his and our favorite group, the Beatles.

We are so grateful to good friends for helping us get this important part of our house "all together now".

CHAPTER 9: FUN AND GAMES AROUND OUR COURT

Last Thursday, which happened to be St. Patrick's Day, a couple of our wonderful neighbours invited us to a St. Patrick's Day party at their home just up the street. There was plenty of green beer and lots of wine. There must have been 20 of us, all from the same street plus a few other friends and family members.

There must have been about five guitars around the room, which were being picked up occasionally, along with a few dozen sheets of Irish music that most of us joined in on and had an absolute riot with. Let me tell you that I can't carry a note and most of the partiers admitted the same but we were all hooting and laughing with the likes of "When Irish Eyes are Smiling" and "The Unicorn" with Tom and a few others accompanying on guitar.

When the party seemed like it was starting to thin out, I noticed a few guitars also slipping out. I will just remind you here briefly that before I had this sickness, I was in a band with some buddies and we were playing rock music like there was no tomorrow. I played lead guitar with my Fender Stratocaster and now, since my sickness, I am not able to form the chords anymore because of my left arm and hand paralysis. At the party, I looked over at the son of our gracious hostess, Tom, who certainly was quite proficient on the guitar and was knocking out some familiar Irish tunes, and I got him to hold the left end of the guitar while I took up a pick and began to strum the right end. Of course, I have stated before and I keep telling my therapists that my ultimate goal is to get my left hand functional again and be able to make my favorite sounds with a guitar once more. So, Tom and I were belting out a few chords and songs and I can tell you that it almost sounded like we knew what we were doing.

I can't tell you enough how therapeutic it was for me to be participating in music and helping make those sounds again. It was almost like a dream come true, even though my left hand isn't quite functional yet! I thank you, Tom for this opportunity! It was a riot!

CHAPTER 10: WITH A LITTLE HELP FROM OUR FRIENDS

Today was a special day. Our good friend, Drew, who we met for the first time at our Taoist Tai Chi Health Recovery week in Orangeville in September, came to visit and stayed overnight after a long trip from his home in the Niagara region. We are so lucky to have met the most wonderful people at the Taoist Tai Chi Health Recovery weeks we have been attending since September. The experiences have been truly refreshing and enlightening as all the encounters have been with very intelligent people and every conversation over lunch is always truly educational and inspiring.

Hélène made a wonderful Chinese meal for us for supper as she has recently been making quite often with her wok. Corey and I have been enjoying these meals so much almost every day. She is such a great cook and we are usually known to have seconds and thirds. Actually, I'm lying! This night, I had four servings of this extremely healthy meal of vegetables, brown rice, Thai noodles, chicken and succulent shrimp. For dessert, Hélène served us fresh fruit and vanilla yogurt. Mmmm! The entire meal was delicious. There wasn't much to clean up, much to Corey's delight that evening as he customarily cleared the table for us.

Drew and Hélène and I had a pleasant visit, talking about many things including Drew's and my experiences with our strokes, our former professional lives, Hélène's experience and perspective of living through my stroke and the profound knowledge and the experience she has gained through getting to know other stroke victims and some M.S. patients.

I have to admire and am very proud of my wonderful wife, Hélène, for many reasons. For one thing, she is extremely intelligent, always demonstrating her expertise in grammar and spelling, including her acute knowledge of current events and entertainment, including actors, actresses and other worldly entertainers. She can rifle off names, birthdays, ages, relationships, not to mention her gift for remembering phone numbers!

Today was an absolutely gorgeous day, typical of just how superb this past summer has been. It was about 26º C, sunny with just a little wind. It was another day for t-shirts and shorts. We have just been so lucky this summer. Very few days have been too hot and most days have been comfortable enough to please most anyone. We actually only reluctantly closed our pool yesterday, October 8. Our gracious and always helpful neighbour, Dave, came over and helped Hélène pull the cover over the pool and tighten the securing wire. Dave gave his usual advice on each of the techniques of a typical pool closing and Hélène administered the $75 in pool closing chemicals she had purchased yesterday, a small price to pay considering the quality of the water and the enjoyment we derived from the pool all summer. We never lost control of the quality of our water even once all summer, which can be a rarity as you would know if you have ever owned a pool.

Drew is an incredibly intelligent man. He is able to speak articulately on nearly any topic. He is particularly and acutely knowledgeable on PC and general computer applications. He was able to speak of and just generally help me on a few aspects of my PC's performance, giving me solid advice and tips on many of my existing computer applications and its installed software.

We both have the same Zire 72 Palm Pilots and he was able to give me infinite guidance and assistance with many of its features and characteristics. In a few short hours, I was able to learn and eventually derive considerably more benefits and service from this amazing little but powerful device. We worked until late into the evening with Drew finding many performance enhancing opportunities with my PC. I was delighted! My PC was running like a top when we finally wrapped up at about 12:00 am. I was ecstatic but we had had enough. Time for bed. Poor Drew. He took his dog for a last midnight walk, I let Cooper out for a final pee and Drew slid his 6'2" frame into the computer room's small day bed and I snuggled into bed with Hélène, taking no more than about five minutes to fall into a solid slumber for the night.

Drew and I had a lengthy and soulful discussion that night about our experiences with our strokes. Drew's eloquence enabled him to speak extremely accurately and knowledgeably about his overall experience and the disaster of having had a stroke. His experience gelled well with mine and I believe we were both able to provide each other with assurances and advice that should help us to understand and, in some cases, make additional decisions on what some of our logical and desirable next steps in our recovery plans and attempts should be.

A few days later, Drew and I were chatting on the phone. You have to realize that something as simple as a friendly, social phone conversation for stroke survivors is a serious, complex matter for them to undertake, considering our brain surgeries and short-term memory challenges. Well, this time I got up the will and determination to look up his phone number in my email address book and call him. Drew and I shared our latest activities.

Drew told me that he has been going to the YMCA near his home lately and he advised me of his latest milestone! He told me that he had actually been able to break into a run a little bit. I am so proud of him. That is such a big step in the grand scheme of things, considering his balance issues and difficulty walking. And I told him of a major milestone for me. Well, last night, we were entertaining a couple who had joined us for a BBQ. We had gone in the pool and I prepared, as I usually did, to attempt to swim a couple of laps. I had gone in a few times last year after my wife had raised the water temperature to my comfort zone of about 95ºF. After getting in the water and swimming the first couple of laps with Hélène and Paul (Joan isn't a swimmer), I was soon swimming a few laps without my life-jacket, an absolute first for me - actually, pretty much almost a miracle. Well, so this week marked a couple of major milestones for Drew and me. I honestly cannot wait for what's going to come next! Don't get me wrong. I am far from being a Mark Spitz! My left leg is certainly still paralyzed, but my hip seems to work somewhat and I can execute a reasonably normal swim kick, but my left hand and arm are totally flaccid and do not participate at all in my swim attempts. So I am resigned to swimming – usually – with a life jacket unless there is extra help in the pool with us.

When anyone has had a stroke, the mind is the most affected. A "Brain Attack" is no trivial matter. Concentration, decision-making and thought processing cause considerable discomfort in the head. In my case, when I exercise the cranial components, my head tightens from my forehead to the back of my skull to the degree that I just want to fall to the ground and roll over and over and cry and scream. Fortunately, my physical disability and remaining logic prevent me from attempting such a desperate action. Yet, my skin feels as though it is so tight and too small for my body. Tonight, upon returning home from a BBQ at the home of our dear friend Marcela and her husband, Nick, where we were treated to a wonderful dinner of chicken, some wine and salads, I was undergoing a pretty serious bout of thalamic pain. My thumb and index finger were tingling and screaming like one's tongue would feel when its tip is touching a 9 volt battery, except they were feeling like they were being charged with the current from a 24 volt battery. So were my toes. I explained to my wife, during this experience, that I was thinking that it was as though the activity of the socializing of the afternoon was stimulating my brain which in turn was sending these pain signals to my extremities. We finally arrived at home and Hélène hurriedly served me my evening's usual concoction of blood pressure and pain medication. After a while, as usual, I didn't feel much better.

CHAPTER 11:   THOSE WERE THE DAYS

While watching one of the best WWII movies I've ever seen, "The Battle of Britain", I was having an attack inside my head that felt like 1,000 bees inside a beehive. The dizziness was so intense that I couldn't sit up straight and I had to close my eyes and pretend I was asleep so that I could ignore the nightmare that was happening. This was to be the "state of the nation" for me for months, even years to come.

At this moment, late Saturday afternoon, I am once more not feeling well. I was feeling the same last weekend and didn't even touch a bite to eat until Sunday. With my head spinning and feeling kind of nauseous, I have been watching my DVD boxed set of "Band of Brothers" all afternoon. I love this and any story about the Second World War. The stories in this boxed set are so realistic and accurate that I feel as though I am really there, actually participating in the battles and raids. The stories are so vivid, I feel as though I am right there defending platoons from certain death in various campaigns. This series is so true-to-life, after all, it is produced by Tom Hanks and Steven Spielberg, so how could it not be a marvelous production? As a matter of fact, I truly wish I had actually been there to participate and contribute.

I am a huge WWII buff and cannot get enough of it, I suppose because my Dad fought in the war and survived. In fact, Mom and Dad met during the war over in England. I am so proud of them and the interesting, valuable lives they had during these important and significant times.

As you read on, you will discover that my racing mind has brought me to one of my favorite topics, which I love and respect so much, because it involved my Dad, who served in the war and of whom I am so proud. I am also so very proud of my Mom who recently passed away and who served as a Women's Division/ RCAF during the War and became a war bride, marrying my Dad back in 1941. In 1943, Mom was recruited by the RCAF. She worked in the Signal Section of the Women's Division of RCAF Headquarters. I hope you are interested in my little piece of WWII here as it is special to me because of my Mom's and Dad's direct involvement which, to me, makes them heroes.

Mom always used to love telling us about the time in 1944 when she was walking in front of a shop in London that had a huge picture window. A German doodlebug flying overhead came down with a huge explosion, smashing the entire window in front of her to bits, fortunately leaving her uninjured as she shopped.

In October, 1943, Dad completed Armoured Corps Officer Training at Sandhurst Military Academy and reported to No. 2 CACRU (Reinforcement Unit for Canadian 2nd Armored Brigade). There were approximately 75 lieutenants waiting to go.

Because Dad had weapons training in 1942, when the Canadians went over to Dieppe, the 2 i/c (Second in Command), Major O'Brien, asked him to take over the Small Weapons Training in early 1943 and share his experience with other ranks who were also waiting to go to Field Units. They were sent out as reinforcements to active units.

After June 6, 1944, Dad begged his O.C. (Officer in Command) to let him go to an active regiment. It was why he had joined the army, why he had gone overseas. The O.C. let Dad go in September, 1944 but it was in October, 1944 that Dad found himself in an Infantry Landing Craft headed for

Dieppe and eventually was sent to the Sherbrooke Fusiliers in a S.C. (Scout Car). When transported to the unit, he did not secure his kit and sleeping bag on the S.C. and said to himself "What a way to start my war field experience!" Even blaming the S.C. driver didn't help.

After the war, Dad and Mom returned to Mom's hometown, Aldershot, England, where they had gotten married and they visited briefly with Mom's family. A few years later, as the war ended, Dad unfortunately had a kidney operation and then retired from the forces as a Captain. Mom and Dad returned to Dad's home in the Eastern Townships in Québec while he recovered from his surgery; then they moved to Montréal where Dad went to Sir George Williams University, graduating with a BA in marketing and of course raising me and my sister and brother. Getting together recently, my brother and sister and I reflected on what a wonderful childhood and parents we had, growing up with many friends, and doing all the crazy things that good friends and loving family do.

I have included this account of some of my Dad's time in the war, in which he describes the circumstances surrounding the picture that appears below. I am only grateful that these men survived and that my Dad has lived to pass on this experience over 60 years later. Talk about being able to have something so special and so important to not only your family but to the world! It makes me so damned proud. In fact, Dad is sitting with me here right now, helping me with some details as I write this story.

The following is the true story by my Dad, Lieutenant Ed Frost, of himself and his crew who were in the Sherbrooke Fusilier Regiment, B Squadron of the 2nd Canadian Armoured

Brigade. Dad found himself and his Sherman Tank troupe in a predicament on February 25/26, 1945. The photo I am referring to shows the men taking a much needed break from an assault in which they were participating in the Hochwald Forest, Germany. The picture shows the four man crew of the tank that led the left flank column approximately 3600 yards forward at night to capture Marienbaum, Calcar, then Xanten, Germany on March 10, 1945. This was the last day of fighting west of the Rhine River. That night, they moved back to the Grosbeck Forest, Holland and on March 18, to the Reichwald Forest, Germany (Siegfried Line) to prepare for the Rhine Crossing with the Canadian Scottish Infantry Regiment.

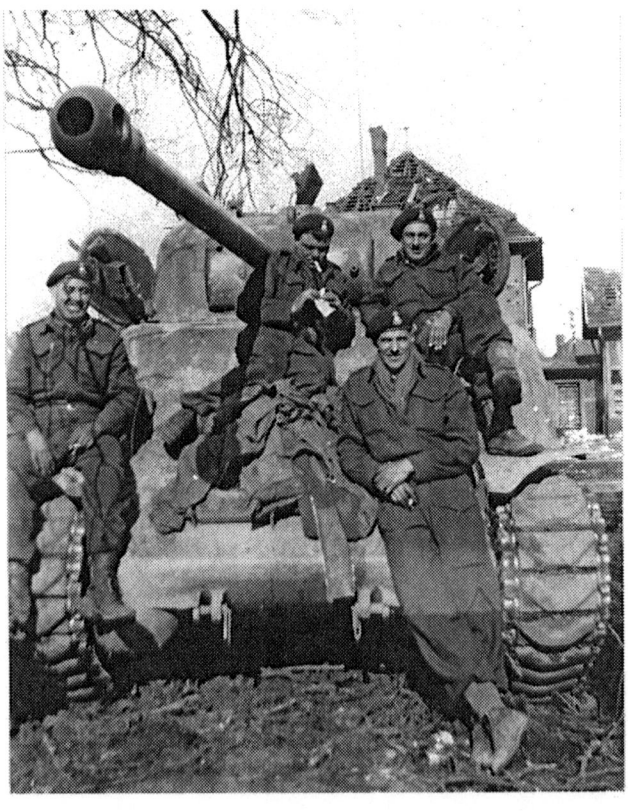

Dad and his tank buddies, Marienbaum, Germany, ca. 1945

The horizon was illuminated with mortar and tank blasts, the fields were thick with shrapnel. We were sure lucky to have made it through the night alive. We were in trouble as there were no gun placements. We thought we had heard a troupe of German infantry running about 200 yards south of us but it turned out to be our own troups reinforcing.

There were three columns in the assault. We had some artificial moonlight that was not too good because of a low ceiling due to a misty rain. The Bofors crew were firing tracer over our heads to help us maintain direction. I had to change tanks twice and we had a third exposure when I had to get out of my turret to push all our kit off the tank because German tracer fire had set it on fire. Our column included flame throwers and flail tanks. The infantry was in Kangaroo tanks toward their assault point.

When daylight came, our three tanks had become very exposed to aggressive German artillery and mortar fire, but we had to stay there all day in case of a German counter-attack with their tanks. We kept zigzagging in the big open farm field so the Jerries couldn't zero in on us.

We had started with four tanks but visibility was so bad that we lost the lead tank in a huge tank trap about 500 yards into no man's land. I fortunately had a Browning M.G. (machine gun) mounted on my lead tank. I took it with me over to the only other tank with a mount for the M.G. Imagine my disgust when I had to leave my machine gun behind when I had to change tanks again due to a faulty radio. I was not able to answer the Squadron Leader's request for "Sit Rep"(situation report)!

I did, however, make a point of ensuring that all my men made it out of there alive.

I was thankful for my Gunnery training and experience as we blasted our way to the objective by use of .17 pdr H.E. (High Explosives) and M.G. fire on any building or copse of trees that could hide the enemy. We had another exposure defending the tank while we stopped to let the crew replenish H.E. rounds from under the turret floor. I survived because I could duck down when Jerry machine gun tracers came our way. We were sure glad it was dark!

I can still hear our Squadron Leader's voice calling for "Sit Rep" every time we stopped!

To this day, I still thank my Troupe Sergeant, Samborne, for protecting my tank's rear exposure for all 3,600 yards, and I thank the Lord our progress was fast enough that the enemy was unable to organize an 88mm defense.

I would be unfair to record this action and not acknowledge the good work of my Radio Operator and Squadron Leader, who served so well loading the heavy 17 pound shells, as he and the Gunner replenished the H.E. load under the turret floor.

SECTION SEVEN – LIFE GOES ON

CHAPTER 1:   GET READY, I'M COMING

I have had many friends and have had a lot of fun with them over the years. Since my strokes and subsequent brain surgery, I have had many vivid and surreal dreams. Also, I recently lost my Mom which broke my heart and left me with an empty feeling, especially when I just want to call her and speak to her.

I nearly died during my stroke. I continue to have a yearning to see the people that once meant and obviously still mean so much to me. I feel as though they all can still see me and I know that I will see them again. I look forward to more laughs, hugs and more good times with them. Please get ready, folks, because I'm coming!

Throughout the course of my life, I have lost a few good friends and family members. About five and a half years ago, I lost my best friend, Dave M., to a virus that took him too quickly. I was called by my friends in Ottawa suddenly one day when they told me that Dave was in a coma and that it did not look like he was going to regain consciousness. I immediately flew to Ottawa to be with him and learn what the hell was happening. His partner, some other friends and family and my wife and I maintained a vigil at his bedside until he passed away three days later. It was unbelievable; in fact, it was practically inconceivable. I could not be losing a friend who had been so loyal and relentlessly supportive in everything I did!

Dave made his friends have "professional development days" where he would get a number of us together at the Air

Force "Officers' Mess", of which Dave was a member. We would shoot pool, drink plenty of draft beer at the cheap military 'Mess Hall' prices and talk and share stories of the successes and challenges we had experienced over the previous week at work and any other interesting experiences we had. The conversations were very encouraging and professionally developmental. They were special and important times.

Hélène and I ended up being part of the intimate group of Dave's friends and family that approved "pulling the plug" and witnessed him pass away. I was able to deliver the Eulogy for him at the funeral. That was a very special privilege.

Another very sad occasion was when our dentist, Dave S., passed away. I had gotten to know him quite well and, in fact, he became a good tennis friend later. He was a wonderful man (a 10 on Peter's "0 to 10 customer service rating system"), a good friend, a loving father and a terrific husband. He died at the early age of 39 of pancreatic cancer. Life is simply not fair sometimes.

Hélène and I were very fortunate and honored to have had the opportunity to go out with Dave and his wife, Deb, during his sickness while he was in remission. We went to the Alanis Morissette concert at the Air Canada Centre with them and some other friends, Joan and Paul, and had a most enjoyable evening. I remember thinking at the time how well Dave looked, all things considered. I guess he had gotten a bit of a reprieve at that point. He died less than six months later.

As I mentioned previously, I had two other very good friends who ended their lives by shooting themselves because of frustration and youthful disappointments. They did not know of each other and were from different eras and locations during my youth and growing up.

I am not a religious person but I do believe in and respect the Ten Commandments. I never want to and never have broken one but I do not believe in God. I want to but I want Him to prove Himself and make my and others' sicknesses just go away. From my understanding, He is supposed to be able to do this. Why should I and others have to prove ourselves first? Only He knows but I believe I have proven myself. Did I deserve this fate? Does anyone? I am confident in my convictions and good intentions. I am a good person. What did I do to earn this fate?

As I said earlier, five and a half years ago my best friend, Dave, passed away rather quickly, of unknown causes. Little did I know that I would almost join him some two and a half years later!

Dave's passing was tragic, as he was very popular and thought the world of his friends and would always do anything for anyone. He also was generous to a fault, always being the first to buy a round of beers at the tennis club or at a round of golf and he always remembered his friends' birthdays with a generous gift.

When I received the call from Jean, one of our many good friends in Ottawa, that Dave had taken seriously ill, was unconscious and was not expected to regain consciousness, I nearly went into shock. I had no idea the poor guy was feeling so grim but I knew he hadn't been feeling well since returning from a temporary government assignment in Bosnia. Dave was still living in Ottawa with his girlfriend and life partner, where he and I had been good buddies and had played lots of tennis and golf with a great group of friends. I had moved to Toronto about 7 years previous and was living in a little town north of Newmarket at the time. I immediately made arrangements to fly to Ottawa to see how he was making out. I got to the Ottawa General Hospital the next morning and met his partner, Alena, as well as some of his relatives and went to see Dave in his comatose state. It was so sad. We talked to him, all the while not getting any response. Eventually, the doctors advised us that there was no sign of life possible for poor Dave and that the life support equipment should probably be disconnected. Let me tell you how traumatic that was for everyone.

Hélène and our boys drove up the next day and I told her the bad news. She too was shocked and very sad. As she said at the time, how could she not love someone who loved her man so much? The following day, we met with the doctor and made the necessary arrangements. We brought Alena's son, David, as well as our two boys in to say goodbye to Dave. Alena's youngest, Danny, had opted not to go as he wanted to remember Dave the way he was when they had last seen each other.

Afterwards, I drove all three boys to David's father's house where Danny was waiting for them. I then returned to the hospital just in time to say my own goodbye. That weekend, while having breakfast over at Alena's, we started making calls and making arrangements for an appropriate funeral service for Dave. We contacted a reasonably accessible funeral home and went over to coordinate the arrangements. Many guests came to the funeral home the night before the funeral to pay their respects. The funeral was nice and special, as nice as something like that can be. The internment was arranged for the following Saturday.

Here is a chronology of the events surrounding this profound loss in my life:

August 30, 2000 (Wednesday) - at 5:45 pm, I was called to Dave's bedside with his family and close friends. I immediately booked a flight to Ottawa for 6:40 am the next day.

August 31, 2000 (Thursday) - I flew to Ottawa. A few of us stayed at Dave's bedside most of the day. He was unconscious the whole time. We never were able to talk to him.

September 1, 2000 (Friday) - We spent a sad day at the hospital. Hélène and the boys drove up to Ottawa that evening.

September 2, 2000 (Saturday) - We agreed with the doctors to have Dave's life support equipment disconnected. Dave passed away.

September 3, 2000 (Sunday) - Alena, Hélène and I made the funeral arrangements. I started to write the eulogy for Dave at Alena's.

September 4, 2000 (Monday) - At 7:00 pm, we attended a visitation at the funeral home.

September 5, 2000 (Tuesday) - At 12:00 noon, Dave's funeral took place. Afterwards, friends and family were invited back to Alena's for a wake. At 12:00 midnight, Hélène, the boys and I returned to Toronto.

September 6, 2000 (Wednesday) - Hélène and I returned to work.

During the funeral service, as Dave's best friend, I delivered a eulogy befitting the relationships Dave had had with many friends and loved ones. Our friend Denis had prepared a CD as a tribute to Dave, which contained the text of the eulogy and a number of Dave's special and favorite tunes, which were played during his funeral.

Here, for your reading pleasure, are some of the stories that appear on Dave's Tribute CD.

CHAPTER 2:   THE CREEK

It was not uncommon for any of us to lose a few golf balls, either over the fences and out of bounds, or more frequently, in the water! My dad would always supply Dave and me with golf balls whenever he saw us as he enjoyed supporting us in our efforts at developing our skills at the game! In reality however, while I suppose we truly did try to improve our mastery (or lack thereof) of golf, it was fortunate we never did have to actually pay for our golf balls.

We were out at the Canadian Golf Club just to the south of Ottawa one day. We were Nigel, Dave, Mike, Hugh, Bernie, John, me, etc., enjoying a fine sunny day on the course instead of at work. After a few holes and having experienced Mike's "running drive" a few times, we (Dave and I were sharing a golf cart) found ourselves at the edge of a creek where my ball had rolled in. Determined not to treat my dad's generosity and thoughtfulness irresponsibly, we were making a concerted effort to retrieve my ball.

I could see my golf ball in the water a few feet from the edge of the fairway. Not having a "ball retriever" in my arsenal, with Dave standing near me to spot the ball, I asked him to hang on to my arm while I leaned in with my 7 iron to pull the ball closer. DUH!

Of course, Dave was quite willing to oblige and held my arm while I stretched over the water and made contact with the ball, and as I pulled it closer, HE LET GO OF ME!

Well, it was obvious to those around us what had happened, as I screamed at him while I stood, in my golf shoes and socks, in water up past my knees. His friends knew, all too well, his famous "Cheshire Cat grin"!

CHAPTER 3: THE GOLF CART

One thing about spending time with Dave…you never knew what was going to happen next.

And the competitive spirit was evident in everything we did, whether trying to score well in a game (any game) or simply trying to outdo one another. Of course, this nearly always resulted in a laugh!

Now, having earlier been nudged into a creek along the fairway while trying to retrieve my golf ball, of course I was waiting for my opportunity. However, to have immediately attempted any form of revenge would have kept Dave on constant alert and most certainly wouldn't have allowed me to use the element of surprise which, with Dave, one needed if satisfaction was to be attained.

So, about three holes after my "soaker", I was driving our golf cart down the middle of the fairway of a long par 5, thinking all the time about an appropriate opportunity for retribution. I believe Dave was heavily into a philosophical tirade about the merits of professionalism or the gross incompetence of the public or private sectors. I slowly started to make my move.

I argued with Dave about how, on Fridays, there were never any cars in the parking lots of federal office buildings. He lambasted me back on how private companies flushed profits down the toilet with extravagant expense accounts and other such wasteful policies. As the conversation intensified and Dave sipped on a beer he got from the pretty refreshment cart girl, I craftily edged our golf cart over toward the gradual bank of the pond along the fairway.

When we were only a few feet away, I turned the cart towards the bank and began to drive with the passenger-side tires a few inches in the water. Soon the water was coming up over the open side of the cart and onto the floorboards. Dave, his eyes opened wide laughing at whatever the hell I thought I was doing, lifted his feet and balanced his still almost full beer. At that moment, the cart still moving…I JUMPED OUT!

Well, the sight that ensued was priceless. The cart coasted another few feet or so into the pond and Dave, thinking quickly as he always did, jumped into the water, soaked half way up his thighs, his beer long lost, and stood holding the cart from tipping right over into the pond. Cursing, laughing and screaming at me to give him a hand, I was not too helpful, rolling over in a fit of laughter safely way up on dry land.

The golf cart was saved. His pants, socks and shoes, however, were another story!

CHAPTER 4:   THE ATM

Many times, Dave would arrange for his colleagues at work to meet with his tennis buddies and he would take us to the Air Force Officers' Mess on Nepean Street where he was a member. It was a super spot to go because the beer was cheap and there were pool tables. It was a further example of how special he considered his friends because he merely wanted to spend and share quality time with us.

We would start there right after work and have a few games and beers. The beer was very cheap and we could talk about our eventful or stressful week on the job, making other people look good or rich while we drove the business. Mediocre pay-cheques are tolerable when one feels like they were solely responsible for the success of our organizations. A little self-indulgence and the occasional respect and recognition from our superiors enabled us to stick with the program! We also motivated ourselves where other stimuli were not available. We called these…*"professional development days"*!

So after about two or three hours of priming ourselves at the mess' economy rates, we would head to the next venue. Usually live entertainment was the goal or perhaps the Lieutenant's Pump on Elgin Street where we could be obnoxious playing pool, shuffleboard or darts. However, after paying for umpteen pitchers at the mess, we usually needed to visit an ATM.

This particular night, we left the mess with the intention of hitting the Lieutenant's Pump next. Someone drove us to Elgin Street and parked. Some went immediately over to the bar. Dave and I and a colleague of Dave's (someone please tell me who he was, I forget…apologies) went to the ATM across the street from "The Pump".

I recall that Dave used the machine first. Then, when he was done, Dave, in his customary competitive style, began to jump and demonstrate how he could hit the plastic honeycomb lighting ceiling panels with his head!

Not to be outdone, once I was finished with my transaction, I tried to do the same. I was barely successful. Dave was gloating about his superior dexterity with his usual prowess. Once he retrieved his cash, it was his buddy's turn. He was a few inches shorter than we were, but he tried a few times. Dave, laughing at the inadequacy, while a fourth attempt was being made, grabbed his buddy's elbows during a leap and proceeded to RAM his head through the plastic panel, spreading bits all over the floor of the ATM lobby. Good thing in those days they had not yet installed surveillance cameras!!

Dave's poor buddy barely escaped major head injuries, should a support beam or sprinkler pipe have been concealed by the panel. Once again, hoots and tears of laughter were shared for years after this event.

CHAPTER 5: THE CLUBS

Dave was a perfectionist! And, like most of us, he took great pleasure in getting a good deal...on anything!

Dave was not afraid to spend money however. He liked to have nice things and was generous to a fault. When we were beginning to become more and more interested in the game of golf, Dave wanted to get himself a very good set of clubs. He was aware of a certain individual who had a good reputation for making custom sets for a good price. Dave placed an order.

Finally, a few weeks later, the clubs were ready. Dave picked them up and I think we took the following Friday off work to try them out. Over the next couple of months, Dave got in quite a few games as he increased his interest and skill at the game. By the end of the summer, Dave and his friends had played many games. One thing we all knew was that Dave had a terrific amount of power and could always hit the ball farther than most others. Most golfers know that with a slice, that was not always a good thing. However, that would not deter Dave from attempting to drive the green on most holes.

Soon, it was becoming apparent that an interesting phenomenon was occurring. It seemed that, on shots where most of us would use a 5 or 6 iron, Dave was using a 7, 8 or 9. The usual rules of thumb for club selection did not work for Dave. He always (and had us convinced too) attributed this to his amazing power. It seemed to make sense. But as time wore on, Dave was finding that on his approach shots, he was frequently hitting OVER the green.

Then one day, while our foursome and the ones in front and behind us were chatting and jesting, awaiting our turns on the tee, Dave looked intently at the head of one of his irons, the 7 iron I think. He passed it over to us to have a look. He asked to see one of ours. He said, "Guys, am I crazy or does my 7 iron look a little unusual to you?" We all took a look. Then we inspected his 8, 9 and then even his 6 iron. Before long, we were hooting and bellowing with laughter!

It seemed that the fame, reputation and credit that Dave had earned for his awesome power that flew the ball further than any of us, was only partly due to his power in hitting the ball. It was now obvious to us that what was sending his ball further on all his shots was that he swung his clubs so hard and usually struck the ground causing the loft on each iron to decrease, that his pitching irons looked and performed more like 2 or 3 irons!!!!

Dave finished the season with those clubs…and purchased a new set the following spring!

(Note: For those of you who do not understand this story, please consult your closest golfer-wanna-be!)

CHAPTER 6:   THE POOL TABLE

A true friend is someone who will do anything for his friends. Dave was just this to certain people.

It had become routine procedure for the Monday night tennis league at the OAC to go upstairs for beer and wings after our showers. There, we would talk about the games of the evening, play Trivial Pursuit and usually verbally abuse each other. It was a continuation of our competitiveness.

There were ten of us who played on three courts each Monday evening from 6:30 to 8:30 pm and then we would be upstairs in the restaurant enjoying a meal until about 10:00 pm. Dave had negotiated the "permanent" private court time and we truly had a quality league of selected tennis players whose skills and personalities fit/made the group. Once done in the restaurant, however, it seemed that most of us still had the adrenaline flowing from the hard hitting and stimulating camaraderie. We then would leave the club and go across the street to the Den!

Now, the Den was an establishment that was generally considered as a "Gentlemen Only" type of place. It featured "exotic" entertainment, however was not typical of many less reputable such venues that one would not want to frequent or be seen in. It was well run with a professional ambiance. The management, service and food were excellent and, most importantly, it had eight pool tables! This was the sole reason we went there! Competitiveness (or is that competiveness? as Dave recited many times) was never over until our heads hit the pillows later that evening!

Well, this one typical Monday evening, after we had had our dinner at the club, we agreed to head over to the Den. Most of us went and some had to go home. That night, Pat was the first to arrive!! As is advisable in this busy and somewhat rowdy place, Pat secured a table for us by placing his coins in the slot and racking up the balls for our first game. Pat was pleased with himself. At this point, I believe he walked over to peek at the event on the stage. A few minutes later, he came back to the table to find a 250 lb. long-haired, tattooed motorcyclist enjoying Pat's pre-paid balls.

I remember arriving at this point and walking over to Pat who proceeded to tell me what had happened. I hesitantly but determinedly walked over to the cyclist (and whatever else his occupation/profession might be), his sidekick and an apparent bimbo and told them they were playing on our coins! He grunted something back that seemed to suggest a lack of concern or regard for my comment. Then Dave arrived at the table. What happened next was "classic Dave"!

Dave, in his customary assertive voice, walked over and expressed to the dude that he was using our money and that this was OUR table and would he please place some fresh coins in the table so we could proceed to play! A reasonable request, we thought!

The leather-jacketed thug then stood up in front of Dave and began to express where he wanted to place the pool cue he held in his hand. In a split second, Dave had the man up against the wall, his feet 24" from the floor, holding him up with undoubted determination and once more proceeded to explain how he was out of line! Bouncers converged immediately on the scene and I guess we thought we were all scheduled for a quick escort to the parking lot. However, our regular well-dressed tennis group was always respected by the establishment and, fortunately, they recognized the irresponsible behavior of the thug and threw him out, apologizing to us for the inconvenience caused.

Dave's virtue and morality prevailed once more!

CHAPTER 7:   THE DRYER

The joys of home ownership include making enhancements over the years to make one's home more comfortable and to increase its value. Dave loved to use tools and develop his own handiwork in increasing the value of his home. Sometimes he consulted with other experienced people to get tips on how to proceed. Sometimes he didn't!

Dave actually did an excellent job rearranging things in his home. Not pictures or furniture, but walls,…floors,…windows…and stairs! Serious stuff! Everything he did made the house look better than what it was before. After the upstairs had been worked on, and beautifully done I might add, he started on the basement. The project included a laundry room, a bathroom and a cozy recreation room.

Once more, the final product was beautiful: fine pine walls, three-piece charming lavatory and functional laundry room with lots of needed shelving and storage space.

There was one problem!

One day, the dryer quit! After a few unsuccessful attempts at engineering a technical repair (Dave was trained and skilled at avionics…not electronics!), it was decided that a new dryer was required. This was when the problem was discovered. Not initially detected by the naked eye, it became apparent that the dimensions of the dryer exceeded the clearance of the stairway opening leading from the basement. The carefully crafted doorways and jams of beautiful solid pine would not allow initial attempts to get the lifeless dryer up the stairs.

Determined, Dave called on a few friends (Andy, Peter and Clark) to assist in some Kreskin caliber geometric metaphysical manipulation which should have, with careful coaching, enabled us to get the dryer up the stairs and outside the house. This attempt was to no avail.

Not to be deterred, Dave proceeded to the next and obvious (well, to him anyway!) step. Dave disappeared into the well-equipped workshop and soon emerged with a tool of sophisticated purpose and high level training, one of his favorites, a SLEDGEHAMMER!

Well, the sight that was to ensue was one not to be forgotten! It is necessary to point out that the next few moments were advisable to be experienced from a slight distance. Dave proceeded to reconstruct the molecular structure of what was once a shiny, solidly built Kenmore dryer. He proceeded to pound and pummel with inherent brute strength and untiring energy until the virgin-white appliance was indistinguishable from a mangled Tonka toy trodden by a herd of horny hippos!

For the next few minutes, the hammer swung and parts and pieces flew everywhere. In a short while, the dryer was easily carried in pieces up the stairs and outside to the curb.

Well, you can imagine that afterward, we were then able to pause and reflect on the success and determination that Dave had resolved that day. But then there was another problem!

How was Dave to get the new dryer downstairs?

CHAPTER 8: THE BUS STOP

One year, on New Year's Eve, Dave had called me to say he was on his way over to my house for a quick drink after playing tennis at supper hour. He should have arrived at 7:30ish.

At approximately 8:30 pm, he called me from his cell phone or a phone booth…I cannot be sure! He advised me that he was actually on his way over but that he needed a hand from me right away before he arrived. He told me to meet him a few blocks from my house. I immediately drove to the intersection to which he had instructed me to go. What I found was nearly indescribable!

As I arrived on the scene, there was Dave's 4 x 4 delicately pirouetted on an OC Transpo bus stop bench! The bench apparently was what had stopped him while in the middle of a few 360º spins he had skillfully maneuvered down the boulevard. I am not sure if the spins had been voluntary.

We commandeered at least four people to unhitch the vehicle, some of whom, had they been along a few minutes earlier, may have been involuntary direct participants in Dave's "Evil Knievel" stunt!

CHAPTER 9:   THE TAXI

The buddies never really ever expressed any desire to enter politics. This day, Dave surprised us!

Dave preferred Japanese cars or American/Canadian 4 x 4s. At the time, Dave was driving one of the three 4 x 4s that he had owned within a relatively short period (about three or four months).

One afternoon, he was on a particular errand and he found himself at the corner of Sussex and MacKay in New Edinburgh. This was only a few hundred meters from the Prime Minister's residence. A city bus was parked in the intersection, blocking his view to the left of the oncoming two-lane city traffic. So, Dave edged out!

Usually intolerant of less-than-capable urban drivers, he crept out from the intersection to a point where he might see if there was any oncoming traffic. Totally screened by the big bus, he saw a momentary break in the traffic and went for it!

What happened next was spectacular!!!

As Dave veered his vehicle beyond the obstruction of the bus, a city taxi came flying past the bus and struck the nose of Dave's truck, launching the taxi more than 2.5 meters into the air, flipping itself over Dave's hood. The taxi landed a few meters up the street. The hood of Dave's car looked like it had been flattened by a Mac Truck!

The next day, in his usual suppressed melodramatics, Dave told me that his car was in the shop for some badly needed "maintenance". I was not left with the impression that the "maintenance" involved actually "writing off" and replacing the six month old vehicle!!!

It seems that Dave owned three such SUVs in a row that never had time to accumulate any "road wear"!!!

CHAPTER 10:   THE LAWN MOWER

When you have a garage sale, the prime objective is usually to be rid of items that are no longer of use to you and to find a new domain for them to pretend to be of use to. A secondary objective (in fact, in many cases, this actually becomes the primary objective) is to recover some of the initial cost of the investment earlier made in these valuable and once precious trinkets/accessories/must-haves.

One late summer day (August 1990, I believe), we were having a garage sale on my front lawn (advertised jointly by every neighbour on the block). All of Dave's no-longer-desirables had been lugged over the previous evening. Sales began at the crack of 7:00 am Saturday morning and the two finest garage salesmen you ever knew were busy entertaining offers and convincing people that there were no better deals to be had anywhere. Although the whole "garage sale" concept had initially left us with uncomfortable feelings (missed tennis games, golf games and beer and pizza sessions), we actually had fun profiting from the naïve and desperate (we found out later that that is exactly what the experienced garage sale shoppers thought Dave and I were).

As the day drew into the afternoon, we realized we were pulling in a lot more money than originally anticipated. We were amazed at how our precious junk meant so much to some people. Imagine that we could actually get 50¢ for a like-new GE self-cleaning steam iron!

Dave and I had, weeks before, talked about how we both needed new lawn mowers. So the decision was quickly made to go to Canadian Tire before closing at 5:00 pm and make these investments with our huge stash (Dave had hauled in $176 and I had $185). We got this brainstorm at 4:45 pm so we needed to hustle.

A customer then came along and was browsing through our valuables. Less than half of our goods had been taken away so far. He asked how much we would let the lamp go for (marked at $2) and Dave, in his shrewd business-like manner, told him, "We are closed mister. HOWEVER, for $20, you can have EVERYTHING you see that's left here!!!...but you HAVE to take it ALL!"

The dude pulled out his wallet and Dave said, "SOLD!" and we shut the garage door, leaving everything out on the lawn for the guy to figure out how was going to get it all home in his Honda Civic. We then jumped into Dave's Explorer (his first of three he owned over three years…but that's another story) and we sped away to the nearest Canadian Tire store.

Now, those who know where my house was at that time also know that it takes more than 15 minutes to get to Canadian Tire from there. So, with the time constraint at hand, Dave took a route solution that had not been previously navigated. At 4:59 pm, we actually found ourselves in the lane on the opposite side of the divided boulevard, staring across the road at the store whose lights were beginning to be turned out.

A handful of cars remained in the parking lot as the business day was at an obvious close. Dave had his lengthening grass in mind as he made his next move. There was pretty heavy traffic in the boulevard's opposing lanes that were between us and the store's entrance.

Without hesitation, Dave mounted the median with his 4 x 4 and slowly but deliberately edged his way in front of and through the startled traffic…four lanes worth including the right and left turn lanes! He pulled into the parking lot and drove up and over the sidewalk, backing his vehicle to the front doors of the store.

Dave walked into the store as though he was the mortgage holder and to the first clerk we saw, he said, "We're here for our lawn mowers! Do you have them ready for us???"

The startled clerk called for his boss and told him of the request. Dave then told him we had been there earlier, had checked out the options, had now made a decision and a brown-haired, pimply - faced clerk had promised us that the machines would be ready waiting in boxes at the door for 4:30 pm. We even apologized for being a little late.

The manager said that the supposed clerk must have finished work earlier and he had not been made aware of the sale. Detecting Dave's obvious look of dissatisfaction (Dave detested incompetence), he immediately offered us to browse (as he locked the doors) and make our selections. After asking the obvious questions one would ask about a lawn mower (i.e. which one cuts the most grass in the least amount of time?), we made our purchases.

We were soon back home (including picking up a replacement case of beer for the one we exhausted during the garage sale) by 5:30 pm.

SECTION EIGHT – THINGS I'VE TRIED

CHAPTER 1: THE EAGLES' FAREWELL CONCERT AND OTHER DIVERSIONS

I woke up at 6:30 am on Thursday morning, March 30, 2005. It was the morning after the Eagles' Farewell Tour concert which ended up being a fantastic experience. They were so great. Hélène and I have seen a few great concerts together over the years but we agreed that this had certainly been the best.

I could not sleep again after I woke up in the middle of the night so, of course, I got on the computer. As usual, I had many ideas on my mind and I had to get up to get them on paper before I forgot them which, I have to concede, is just the way my mind usually works now. Hélène bought these tickets for me for Christmas and we had been waiting for this concert for three months. The day had finally arrived.

Our trip downtown was quite successful. I say 'quite', because it is not as though I can just take an excursion like that for granted anymore. We are usually in the van and can come and go as we please. I am usually reasonably comfortable mentally and physically. If my head or some area of my body starts to get uncomfortable, at least we know we can always just leave and go home.

Venturing downtown on a fairly long ride on the GO Train is quite an undertaking. Once we leave, we are stuck and there are still a few challenges to anticipate and manage.

For example, I am experiencing considerable pain in my left ear that I have not been able to obtain an explanation for nor do I understand. Also, I get a frostbite sensation in my toes even when riding in a warm train. I have been getting this pain in bed at night also. I just don't understand it because the room and our bed are certainly warm enough and not so cold that my feet would actually be truly cold. However, I do wake up and complain to Hélène and she wraps my feet so that my toes no longer have that frozen feeling and I get comfortable again. I have asked my physiatrist what this pain means because it seems strange. I seem to get it for no specific reason; my toes and fingers just seem to feel so cold that they begin to hurt as though they are frostbitten. I have been told that it is Central Pain and I have read about something like it called Thalamic Pain which is simply part of the neurological recovery from a stroke.

Actually since this experience, I have been to the Dizziness Clinic at Sunnybrook Hospital and I asked the doctor there about the pressure at the back of my head and about my "earache". He explained to me that the pressure is a result of the procedure used to drain the blood from my head after the second bleed. He called this pressure a "post sub-occipital craniectomy headache". He said it is very common following the type of operation I had. In fact, 60% of patients tested following this type of procedure suffered from the same type of pressure symptom. When he looked into my ear, he saw no sign of an infection and told me that it is actually not my ear that is hurting, but my jaw. It is all part and parcel of the same "headache". However, this sensation in my toes is simply excruciating and I want it all to go away. You can read about Thalamic Pain in Section 9, Chapter 2.

Anyway, last night my darling wife and I went downtown to the Air Canada Centre by GO Train which was a huge breaking out for me as it was an attempt at some much desired independence considering the impact of my stroke. I was quite the trooper though, even though my head was thick and congested with many thoughts and I was, yet again, enduring a lot of pain. I was determined to make the trip enjoyable and successful and I think I can truly say that I made it and we had a wonderful time. I did not even have difficulty with the lights or the volume of the music. I thoroughly enjoyed the show, had some popcorn, a couple of beers and a hot dog. It was a successful experiment to get out for such a show and we will certainly do that again. I did consider the ride downtown quite challenging as far as concentration and focus went but I don't think I made any mistakes or errors in judgment although figuring out elevators all the way downtown was quite a challenge and an adventure for Hélène and me.

So, it is now March 26, 2006 and Hélène, Tyler, Corey and I are having supper together to celebrate my birthday. I just got the greatest gift. They gave me the DVD boxed set of the Eagles' Farewell Tour. Wow! I was so pleased. That was such a wonderful concert and I watched the DVD this evening. In fact, it was almost a year to the day since we actually saw the concert live in Toronto – March 29, 2005.

The other thought that I had, which I admit is a little way out there, is along the theme of the sport/game of golf. Last year, I was introduced to wheelchair golf. Golf is a great game that I used to play, although not too avidly. I did enjoy the occasional game with my friends when I still lived in Ottawa. This year, Hélène and I have been talking a bit about her learning the game so that we could both try to enjoy playing it together. I think we will have to get in touch with the Ontario March of Dimes again like we did last year and see if we can get back into a wheelchair golf clinic and take some lessons again. I know that we can always start Hélène into lessons anytime but they are a fair commitment of time and expense. I suppose the priority has to be to try to get me walking and improving as much as I can. Let me tell you that you can plateau in your recovery efforts and, if and when that happens, depression can set in which can keep you from improving any further.

Other inspirations that have had a significant impact on Hélène and me are the Oprah Winfrey and Dr. Phil shows. While millions of viewers tune in to these wonderful talk show hosts and their shows every day, Hélène and I became addicted to them in a different sort of way, different than just becoming exposed to TV shows and deciding to tune in every other day. It was more like we were absolutely SOLD on them!

Hélène had told me about the Oprah and Dr. Phil shows years ago, before my stroke. I never really paid that much attention to them then because I spent any spare time I had on my guitar, playing tennis or renovating our new home. After having my stroke and becoming confined to my hospital bed, Hélène was usually allowed and encouraged by the wonderful staff at my rehabilitation hospital, Bridgepoint Health, to spend as many hours as possible with me. If she wasn't there when I would awake, I would usually cry myself to sleep, so I was so grateful to the amazing staff there for being so understanding and compassionate. That is when I was first exposed to Oprah and Dr. Phil. Gads, we would never miss those shows and we still don't. I'm not exactly sure how this came to be but between Dr. Phil and Oprah's Angel Network and the good news stories they produced, we sure end up shedding many tears together. I guess when you are convalescing, recovering and it seems like all the chips are down, it is only natural that your emotions are close to the surface. I tell you, I have had to learn to manage my tears because, before I was sick, I could never cry.

My wife is an all around intelligent person, so much in tune with what is going on in the world around us and is incredibly astute; she has a knack for remembering telephone numbers, has excellent grammar and spelling skills and knows the names and relationships of all the actors and stars and TV personalities extremely well. Her talent for remembering telephone numbers and dates has turned out to be extremely handy when handling all my doctors' appointments and ordering and managing my $200 worth of prescriptions weekly!

Sunday, September 11, 2005

Life is full of tragedies. Today is the anniversary of 9/11. Yesterday, Hélène and the boys and I drove to Renfrew to see my Dad, my sister, my niece and a couple of my aunts, Auntie Barbara and Auntie Jean. It was so special to see them all, especially my Auntie Barbara and Auntie Jean. I hadn't seen many of my relatives on my dad's side for years, other than at Hélène's and my wedding, when five out of Dad's six sisters were able to share the day with us. Of course, it is much more difficult to see those on my Mom's side because they are all overseas in Great Britain. We want to get over there someday. In fact, we have been talking about it a lot recently.

As I sat in the passenger seat of our van, I was daydreaming and thinking about my life when I was in my twenties and early thirties, which now is about 20 or so years ago.

We had a nice visit yesterday and Dad took us all out for dinner at the end of the day. Unfortunately, I was having a bad day. My head was buzzing as usual and the pressure and the dizziness were so intense that I could barely sit up straight. I really don't get headaches per se but this pressure and buzzing are almost unbearable.

In the last few days, CNN has been continuing its detailed coverage of Hurricane Katrina. Hélène and I find it terribly tragic and emotional to follow these events, especially those now being covered of the rescuing of the pets and various animals. We can't help but shed a few tears every time we see an update. We just find that the world can be so cruel at times, leaving us at the mercy of Mother Nature.

I suppose I feel I am one of those victims - a victim of the grace of God, subject to whatever fate befalls a stroke victim who has survived a life-threatening brain attack!

Of course, my life is so different now. Each waking moment is a painful, mind-twisting exercise that I just wish could be over. Every day, my brain takes me through the moment by moment routines that we all take for granted. I can no longer walk. My left leg and foot are paralyzed and are painfully stiff. My left arm also is totally numb and my hand and fingers have a severe stinging sensation every waking moment. I suppose you could say that I have gotten used to it but when I do think about this affliction, it is heart-breaking. The left side of my face and my lips are numb and my pronunciation seems to drag. Also, I usually gnaw at the inside of my cheeks. My left arm and hand are non-functional. All this crap certainly doesn't make me very happy.

Why the hell did I have to have this stroke anyway? I was enjoying my life and my various activities so much. Four days before this "brain attack" I was performing a great night of rock music.

CHAPTER 2: MY QUEST CONTINUES

As my quest continues for as successful and complete a recovery as possible, I am learning and discovering so much. It is simply impossible to keep up with all the information. I find it an incredible experience even to spend time over lunch chatting with all my Taoist Tai Chi co-participants. Many of them have had their own health issues for years, including stroke, MS, fibromialgia, heart disease and even cancer. Their own desperation and thirst for knowledge about their particular condition have driven them to a life of research. As I am in a similar situation, I find that I too have become driven to a life of information gathering and solution seeking. In most cases, we have heard of someone's success story with certain aspects of their affliction and how they have become obsessed with experimenting with different treatments and medications in an effort to hang on to their last shred of hope. It is one thing to understand and cooperate with traditional Western Medicine, techniques and methods. When one is trying to survive and cope with illness as tragic and serious as stroke, for example, there really isn't anything that isn't worth trying.

Paralysis and the loss of the use of an arm, hand, leg and foot and possible impairment of speech, vision or appearance is not a pleasant consideration so searching for and experimenting with solutions becomes a way of life and an endless and tireless effort for such afflicted individuals. The mystery and education that one can experience and derive from such a quest is exhausting. I find the knowledge out there to be extremely fascinating and, while one doesn't have to be a doctor to be introduced to miscellaneous remedies and potential treatments, it literally becomes a full-time job and certainly is almost equivalent to gaining a university education to try to pull all the information together. The individuals one ends up chatting with over lunch or in the lounge or in a support group are extremely intelligent and possess such a wealth of information, suggestions and ideas. I always have my trusty Palm Pilot close by as I constantly jot down notes and suggestions for follow-up as soon as I get home. I usually can't wait and make limitless entries into my notebook on the drive home.

Today, Thursday, November 10, 2005 was the end of another magical and utterly stupendous week for Hélène and me at the International Taoist (pronounced Daoist) Tai Chi Centre's Health Recovery program where we go for health recovery sessions for a week every month. So far we have attended three such weeks, seeing remarkable improvement and progress in my mobility, balance and stamina each time we go.

A typical Health Recovery week starts with us rendezvousing in the dining room with a number of other Tai Chi co-participants. A typical day starts with Hélène and me and our colleagues, about 32 of us this month, sitting down to a healthy breakfast, professionally prepared by three of our fellow participants. Afterwards, about six of us wash dishes and three of us, including myself, dry them and put them away. I dry from my wheelchair, avoiding having to wash the breakable dishes because I am always afraid that I might drop something. When I dry, it is usually always just aluminum or stainless steel utensils, bowls and pots so there is less risk of me dropping and breaking anything. I can actually fly through the mounds of dishes with my drying partner, quite enjoying the constant chatter and laughs. After all, how many of us really want to take bulk dish drying that seriously, given that we all have more serious things to talk about including our respective aches and pains, as well as our physical challenges and needs. I believe the pain to which I am referring is called Complex Central Pain Syndrome which you can read about in Section Nine. Anyway, I persevere and process dozens of dishes with my partner.

The other two meals are ably prepared by our chef, Alex, who never fails to impress us with his culinary skills. Unfortunately for us, but fortunately for Alex, he will be leaving the centre at the end of December, 2005. His mother has purchased a small restaurant in Dawson Creek, BC and she and Alex will be moving there. Thank you, Alex, for all the wonderful meals. And good luck to you in all your future endeavours!

* As of this writing, Alex has been replaced by Carina, who has proven that she is more than up to the challenge.

After dinner on the first day, we assemble in the lounge for an introductory meeting where the Administrator of the Health Recovery Program, Kelly, covers all the guidelines as well as the schedule for the week and our nurse, Mary, explains the emergency procedures, escape routes in the event of fire, fire "buddies" for those in wheelchairs like myself and we then go around the room introducing ourselves and sharing our respective backgrounds.

Under the watchful and wise eye of our lead instructors and the gentle, conscientious care of the assistant instructors, the miracles continue at Health Recovery week in Orangeville. The breakthroughs have been relentless as the Health Recovery instruction team has continued with their infinite care and guidance to reach milestones in our respective quests for improvement.

I thought I would share with you all a bit of a miraculous discovery that Hélène and I experienced while relaxing one night at HRW. We were sitting in the lounge in front of the fireplace on Tuesday evening and Hélène was giving me a much needed and loving foot massage. It felt so good! I was ecstatic! In fact, it was orgasmic! I was enjoying it so much. Of course, I didn't want her to stop.

What's so unusual about this, you ask? Well, I had to halt my thought process for a moment and think about this. The strange thing was…I was feeling this massage! I was enjoying and actually feeling it. I haven't actually had any sensation at all in my left foot since I had my stroke. It's been two and a half years and I was even feeling these gentle toe kneads and relaxation like one couldn't appreciate enough. After not feeling a stretch or any relaxation in my left foot or left hand for this long, I was experiencing a loosening and relaxation in areas that formerly were just so tight all the time, due to the paralysis I was left with since having to endure the pain and tightness of the tone and spasticity that accompanies a serious stroke. Well folks, there is hope and God is watching over us. I am inspired! This has been a special day and, I believe, a miraculous one.

Hélène lovingly gave me another foot massage Wednesday night and again I felt the enduring relief. So I know I am not just imagining things! It seems as though the hard work and inspiration I have encountered this week at HRW have once more produced significant results and substantial improvement for one, if not a number of the Taoist Tai Chi participants. This week, they have also been working on my walking, my balance and the strength of my legs. I feel as though I have overcome a significant lack of mobility as well as a certain degree of the paralysis I have lived with since my stroke. Also, our lead instructors this week, Dave and John, have guided the assistant instructors in enabling me to experience a lessening of the pain in my left hand. I used to scream in pain whenever I would grasp a parallel or exercise (Don Yu) bar. After massaging and stretching my hand, as encouraged and instructed, I am able to grasp and hold on to the bars without excruciating pain in my knuckles and finger joints. I also deem this a miracle and much appreciated positive progress because I was in so much pain before and it was so difficult to approach or endeavour such helpful workouts because of it.

By Tuesday of this month's Health Recovery week, as the end of our session approached, we had achieved many milestones in some of the recovery strategies that the instructors and assistant instructors tried out with us during these classes. Some of the other instructors and participants celebrated these successes with me. There were lots of hugs and pecks on the cheek to go around. Such is the spirit of Taoist Tai Chi Health Recovery week whenever there are miraculous accomplishments. Mine weren't the only successes to be shared this week. A good buddy of ours, Andy, who has Multiple Sclerosis, went from his motorized scooter at the beginning of the week, to walking while assisted on both sides by instructors, to walking with only one assistant. He is already walking up the long staircase at the back of the practice hall. It is truly inspiring to see his progress. Another participant with M.S., Connie, although confined to a wheelchair for the most part, was walking the parallel bars every day and making significant progress throughout the week. We were all so proud of her and congratulated her. There were lots of hugs and kisses to go around that week, which is usually the norm.

This is our fourth month of coming to the International Taoist Tai Chi Centre for Health Recovery week. Each time we come it is a pleasant experience. We exercise and work very hard and always learn a lot about our bodies and our various afflictions. The participants who come here are usually normal, productive, hardworking individuals and include professionals, labourers, housewives and sometimes even young people who haven't yet charted the course of their lives or determined their career path. The one thing they all have in common is that they all have some kind of physical affliction, whether it is stroke, a heart condition, cancer or multiple sclerosis or any one of a number of other serious ailments; the other thing they have in common is their desire to improve their physical condition through Tai Chi. That is why we all go to *Taoist Tai Chi Health Recovery* classes.

Meal times at Health Recovery weeks are always a stimulating, interesting and enjoyable experience. The food, prepared by the chef, Alex, is always top-rate, mostly vegetarian and is "all you can eat". It is usually Chinese, stir-fry or pasta-oriented.

Today, Thursday, January 12, 2006, Hélène and I just completed our fifth Health Recovery week. We have been fortunate enough to have been able to attend similar weeks for the past four consecutive months. The experience at these week-long sessions is an incredible one. The Taoist Tai Chi Society conducts Health Recovery classes at their local clubs, as well as at their Health Recovery Centre in Orangeville, Ontario. They have an attractive 106 acre property that includes a 30,000 square foot centre that has two practice halls, a spacious and full service dining room, a kitchen and a couple of relaxation lounges. As well, the centre has 40 or so double occupancy bedrooms for stay-over participants.

We always practice lots of Tai Chi, usually starting each day at around 8:00 am, proceeding to the evening, wrapping up at around 9:00 or 10:00 pm. We stop for lunch and supper at 12:00 pm and 6:00 pm for healthy Chinese oriented, vegetarian-based meals, occasionally lightly supplemented with shrimp, tofu, chicken, beef or pork.

Today is Friday, February 3rd and we are once more at the Health Recovery Centre in Orangeville for yet another Health Recovery week, which we attend for a full week every month. Construction of the new **Quiet Cultivation Centre** is proceeding nicely. Four walls are up, the roof is on and the floor has been poured. It is looking like a beautifully-designed, fully functional building. The weather has been favourable this winter, so construction has been able to proceed with little interference from the elements and everything appears to be on, if not ahead of, schedule. We are all excited about it and anxiously awaiting the opening of the **QCC**. The current plans call for an official opening of the practice hall on September 9, 2006, which is International Taoist Tai Chi Awareness Day. At that time, the participants (us) will actually be able to use it for the first time. The official opening of the temple, the largest of its kind in the area, is scheduled for September, 2007.

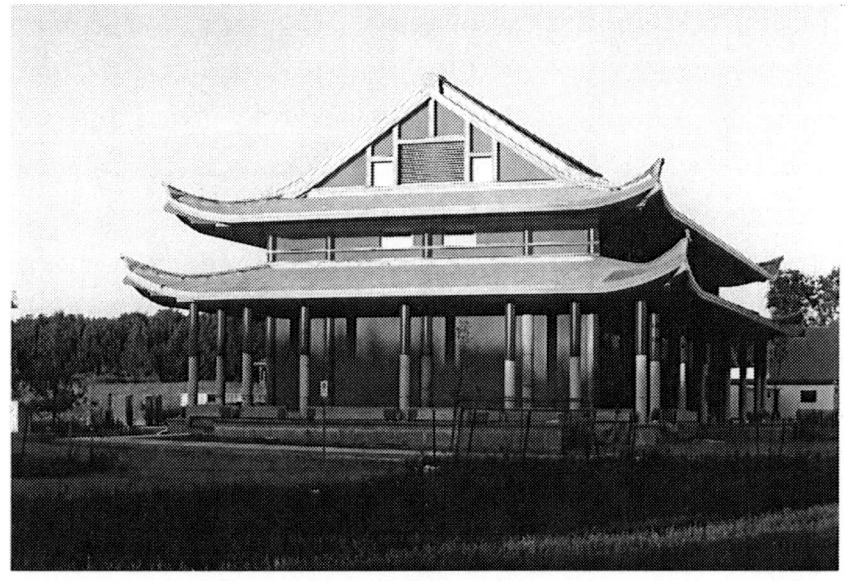

Temple at the QCC, August 2006

The QCC is an extension of the existing facility which is currently comprised of two practice halls, a dining room, a lounge, a kitchen, a wing of bedrooms, some dormitories and some administration offices. Also, on the site is a temple for meditation and paying respect to the late Master Moy Lin Shin, founder of Taoist Tai Chi in Canada, a house for the staff, the Columbarium, a structure that houses the internment remains of a number of the respected deceased of the Taoist Tai Chi Society, including Master Moy and a cemetery which is available to the public.

The QCC is a brand new add-on to the facility. The new practice hall is beautifully designed and will be three times the size of the one we currently use at 10,000 square feet, with a room capacity of 1,000 people!

Tonight, I chatted with my good friends Drew and Andy. They are two very inspirational men. They are enduring their physical problems and represent true survivors. They are both very intelligent men and know so much about their afflictions; Drew is a stroke survivor like me and Andy is handling his M.S. like a trooper. They are amazing examples of strength and fortitude. They both share an incredible wealth of knowledge and information about their illnesses. Together, throughout these very informative and health-associated sessions, we share such a huge human resource of knowledge, hope and encouragement, not to mention, inspiration.

I consider it a privilege to have met such wonderful men that I can call true friends. As part of my book, I thought it would be interesting and inspiring to ask these fellows if they would mind if I conducted a couple of short interviews with them.

One day last November, while at a Health Recovery week at the International Taoist Tai Chi Centre in Orangeville, I asked my friend Andy if he would mind if I conducted a gentle sort of interview with him. I didn't intend or want to interrogate him or probe too deeply into his personal life. It's just that I have always found Andy to be a particularly interesting individual who usually seems to have lots to say. He is very encouraging and inspirational, always providing intelligent and supportive things to say about and for others.

Andy particularly motivates me as I go through my Tai Chi routines, always providing suggestions, wisdom and encouragement. Andy has a great sense of humour and is deeply compassionate toward others. I always learn a lot from him. He has been a decent person to get to know and always offers friendly and humourous companionship when we are in our Tai Chi sessions. He is a true leader and a partner at every encounter and he attributes his personality to always having good people around him.

At the time of our interview, Andy was in the process of wrapping up a photography business in which he had been involved. Although he has been in business for many years and is very good with people, he had decided that his illness would be better managed without the complexity and congestion of the business world. I certainly agreed with him regarding that.

Andy was born in Winnipeg some 51 years ago. He was diagnosed with Multiple Sclerosis 13 years ago and is reminded every day that this is a progressively worsening condition, as opposed to a remitting one, even though, every day, the world seems to be getting closer to finding a cure. At some point, he said, he will probably be forced to take steroids, but for now Tai Chi helps him tremendously, although some months are better than others. October, for example, was a very good month for Andy and the Health Recovery week he spent in Orangeville helped him a lot. By contrast, in November he was much weaker and did not benefit as much from that Health Recovery week as others.

Andy has been happily married to Susan for 30 years and they are the proud parents of two wonderful boys: Chris, who is 26 years old and Adrian, who is 21 years old. Andy considers himself very lucky as he and his wife are best friends. Although Susan sees her friends and she and Andy each enjoy their own time, they frequently go out for dinner, play bridge and relax together.

Andy's "A" type personality makes him a doer rather than a watcher. Through his illness, he has learned what is important in life and believes in 'chilling out'! His bible, so to speak, is the book: "Don't Sweat the Small Stuff" and, shortly after we met, he encouraged me to purchase a copy, which I did. He also subscribes to the philosophy that you have to 'clear the clutter from your brain' once in a while!

Andy also highly recommends taking time every month for a significant, physical tune-up at the Health Recovery Centre!

Drew is another one of those guys that I have been extremely fortunate to meet. Drew was also unlucky enough to have had a near-fatal stroke. Just like me, he is experiencing extreme head and brain trauma and has been enduring his discomfort on a day-to-day basis but he perseveres, with the assistance and encouragement of Taoist Tai Chi.

Drew was born in Northern Ontario some 50+ years ago. He suffered a brain stem stroke, caused by a blockage, about five and a half years ago. Drew is incredibly knowledgeable on the topic of stroke recovery and has been very encouraging to me and other Tai Chi co-participants as he has progressed remarkably through his debilitating illness. I will be eternally grateful for what he has taught me and continues to teach me about this life impacting condition. Drew has progressed through his recovery, which began with him in a wheelchair like me to eventually walking with the assistance of a walker, to now using a cane for balance and to occasionally rest his brain, as he must consciously move his legs. His center of balance no longer functions properly and, as a result, he must balance himself differently. His recovery has been very slow, like mine, and not without a tremendous amount of pain. He must try constantly to improve and keep a positive attitude about his recovery. He sometimes says it is difficult to determine whether he has actually improved or is simply learning to live with his disability.

Drew maintains that his biggest challenge has been overcoming the balance issue and combating the fatigue he feels on a daily basis. Another challenge he faces is the fact that the people around him don't understand his "invisible" disability, being as it is an internal one. The damage to his brain that was caused by the stroke has not interfered with his intelligence, but only with the way in which he processes his thoughts. Things move a bit slower now.

Drew started practicing Taoist Tai Chi in May, 2004. Like me, he has tried alternative medicines, which for the most part have made a difference in his recovery. He is thankful that he did not listen to his doctors, who tended to be somewhat negative as far as his prognosis was concerned. They basically told him to just get used to his *new normal*. "NOT!!!" says Drew. If he had listened to them, Drew maintains he would not have made the remarkable recovery he has made so far. I am so proud of him. He inspires me.

The International Taoist Tai Chi Society has clubs in most major cities around the world including, in Canada: Montréal, Québec; Ottawa, Ontario; Calgary, Alberta; Vancouver,

British Columbia; Winnipeg, Manitoba; Edmonton, Alberta; as well as major cities in the U.S., Europe, the United Kingdom, Australia and New Zealand, Latin America and the Caribbean. We have had the pleasure of meeting and making special and wonderful new friends from many of these places over the past several months. The International Taoist Tai Chi Centre and the Health Recovery Centre are in Orangeville, Ontario (where we go). In addition, there are National Tai Chi Centres in Colchester, United Kingdom; Łódź, Poland; Tallahassee, Florida; Mallorca, Spain; and Rotorua, New Zealand. We plan to go to the Health Recovery Centre every month because it has been so beneficial for me and it is also remarkably rewarding and beneficial for Hélène. After Hélène had been going to the classes with me for about three months, she no longer experienced any of the arthritis or tendonitis pain that she had suffered from prior to discovering this wonderful art.

Taoist Tai Chi is something special that we have discovered and it is truly amazing. We heartily recommend it to anyone, even if they are currently reasonably healthy anyways and just want to maintain their health. For more information on this incredible art, you can look it up under their website www.taoist.org

This endless quest of ours is so interesting and fascinating. There is usually no one specialist who is funded, capable or willing to research and dig into the endless possible solutions, aids and resources to help and improve the wellness of a stroke (or other such afflicted) victim. For example, for months, I underwent physiotherapy at the local hospitals and rehab centres. As I lay in my hospital bed, surrounded by the most qualified and wonderful doctors and best-intentioned nurses and personal service providers in my new ever-prevailing state of paralysis, tone and spasticity, I wondered how much recovery I could reasonably expect to achieve. I wondered if I was even supposed to eventually walk out of there and whether my curved and tightly clenched left hand was ever going to form a G-chord on my guitar again. There certainly were many reality checks and moments when I lacked hope and I would cry and acknowledge to myself that what I was seeing in my current crippled state was all that I was going to get. While this was discouraging, I was learning that part of my therapists' responsibilities was to provide honesty and frankness and not set expectations too high because obviously they could end up with barrages of "You promised me" and "What's next?" and "Why am I not better?" and "When am I going to be able to walk out of here?"

True, there are some traditional and common treatments, such as Western prescription medicine and therapies that we can expect from our local physicians and specialists but the results are usually limited and quite predictable. While under their complete care and mercy, you just can't help but think that they could be perhaps just a little more compassionate and sensitive to your vulnerability, dreams, thoughts and wishes.

In this search for relief and improvement, we have discovered Taoist Tai Chi. This martial art has given me hope, strength and resilience. About two years ago, Hélène, Corey and I went to the Canadian National Wheelchair Tennis Championships in Stoney Creek, Ontario (near Hamilton). We had never even heard of this sport, let alone seen it, so we were naturally curious. While we were sitting courtside, a young woman approached us whose name was Leigh. She was the Coordinator of a program called "Bridging the Gap" which is sponsored by Ontario Wheelchair Sports.

Leigh asked me several questions about my condition, my life, my activity level and what types of activities I had tried. She then asked me whether I had ever tried Tai Chi. I admitted that, no, this was not something I had tried or even really knew anything about. In fact, at the time it didn't strike me as something I would be interested in trying either! Well, Leigh persisted, thank God! She asked whether I would mind if she talked to a woman she knew about me. The woman's name was Assunta. I told her I would be willing to try anything if there was a chance it might help.

Leigh contacted Assunta, who graciously offered to meet me halfway between her home and ours. A date and time were set for our meeting at the Markham Taoist Tai Chi club. Well, let me tell you – Assunta changed my life! She and I spent the better part of two hours together, while she showed me how I could do some of the moves from a chair. Actually, the first thing she did was get me out of my wheelchair and into a regular chair. This was the first time I was sitting in anything other than my wheelchair in over a year.

Assunta is an attractive, petite woman who has Parkinson's Disease. To combat her affliction, she discovered and has been practicing Taoist Tai Chi for over 20 years and has become an instructor, helping and encouraging many other people to do the same. Assunta is one of those people that everyone knows when you mention her name. And everyone loves her!

Thanks to Tai Chi, Assunta is the only member of the Parkinson's Society who continues to take public transit unassisted. She is quite an inspiration. She is very knowledgeable about Taoist Tai Chi, having learned the art and been trained directly by Master Moy Lin Shin himself.

Together, my wife and I have learned and worked hard at learning the 108 moves in a Tai Chi Set, which has allowed us to enjoy and derive health and wellness benefits that we never thought possible. It certainly doesn't even compare to any acknowledged treatment by Western medicine and practices. The thing is, Tai Chi works! It gives you hope, encouragement and faith. Even my wife is enjoying the improvement to her fitness level that has become so important to both of us. Her health and wellness are a necessary part of being able to be my full-time caregiver. She has to draw upon her own energy reserves in order to successfully lift and transfer me from my bed to my chair and to tug and pull at my paralyzed limbs in order to provide me with the daily stretching exercises that are a mandatory part of my routine. Taoist Tai Chi is helping her establish and maintain the strength she needs to move and stretch my 185 lb (85 kg) bulk. It also provides us with the mental stamina that a couple has to share and endure together when faced with such challenges.

Taoist Tai Chi is a form of Tai Chi developed by Master Moy Lin-Shin that he started teaching to a handful of students in Toronto, Canada after moving there in 1970. Now, some 36 years later, the Society now counts approximately 40,000 members in 26 countries worldwide.

Master Moy, who was a Taoist Monk, modified the orthodox Yang style Tai Chi Chuan form, integrating it with his knowledge of other internal arts, such as Lok Hup Ba Fa. One of Master Moy's main teachers was Leung Jee-peng

(Liang Tzu-peng) (1900-1974), an instructor in Lok Hup Ba Fa and other arts from the Ching Wu Martial Arts Academy in Shanghai. Master Moy de-emphasized his new form's connection to martial art training, thereby emphasizing the non-competitive, low impact nature and form of his style of teaching.

There are specific differences in movement which distinguish Taoist Tai Chi from other styles of Tai Chi. Limbs are extended to the fullest extent of their range of motion, providing a stretch for tendons and ligaments throughout the body which is felt to be beneficial for health. In addition, emphasis is placed on rising and sitting, which helps develop balance and leg strength, and helps the practitioner achieve stretch in the lumbar vertebrae and the tendons and ligaments of the pelvis. However, the main differences go well beyond the mere visual aspect. The goal of practising Taoist Tai Chi lies not in perfecting external forms or achieving self-defence skills, but the recovery of lost health in the holistic sense.

The way Taoist Tai Chi is taught differs from that of many other schools in that all instructors are volunteers. In order to become a volunteer instructor, one has to express the desire to do so and be able to show the elements of the form to new students. In addition, there is no "book" from which you can find out everything there is to know about this form of Tai Chi. Everything there is to learn is passed on by word of mouth and by example. A learning instructor is required to attend a number of workshops and should conform to and live by what Master Moy called Eight Heavenly Virtues: a Sense of Shame, Honor, Sacrifice, Propriety, Trustworthiness,

Dedication, Sibling Harmony, and Filial Piety. An instructor should therefore also be a role model to his students.

'Taming the heart' expresses the spiritual aspect to Taoist Tai Chi training.

Master Moy taught that the way to tame the heart is through selfless service and dedication. For this reason, there is great emphasis on volunteerism within the Taoist Tai Chi Society, not only as a way to accomplish tasks of the moment, but as a method of training as integral to the development of good health as any physical exercise.

The prime spiritual aspect of Taoist Tai Chi is the adoption of a spirit of self-sacrifice, generosity and the elimination of self-centredness. Taoist Tai Chi is meant to be taught and practised in a spirit of compassion and service to others.

CHAPTER 3: THE BASIC PRINCIPLES BEHIND TCM

Yin and Yang

Yin and Yang is an important and fundamental concept in Traditional Chinese Medicine.

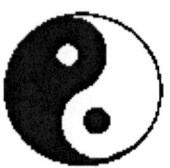

The Chinese character for Yin translates literally as the 'dark side of the mountain' and represents such qualities as cold, stillness, passive, dark, interior, below, front and so on.

The Chinese character for Yang translates literally as the 'bright side of the mountain' and represents such qualities as warmth, activity, light, exterior, above, back and so on.

TCM views the body in terms of Yin and Yang aspects. The healthy state is characterized by a dynamic balance between the Yin and Yang aspects of the body and, by implication, an unhealthy state is characterized by some imbalance between the Yin and Yang of the body.

Excess of Yin - will be characterized by extreme cold symptoms.

Excess of Yang - will be characterized by very full heat symptoms.

Relative Deficiency of Yin - will be characterized by internal heat and lethargy symptoms.

Relative Deficiency of Yang - will be characterized by general coldness and lethargy symptoms.

Yin and Yang exist in dynamic equilibrium; an ideal balance state of health.

Acupuncture is a form of treatment in TCM. The Chinese word for Acupuncture is Zhen Jiu. Zhen means acupuncture and Jiu means moxibustion. Acupuncture is the insertion of hair-like needles into points on the body. These points are located and join together in 'channels' or 'meridians', along which Qi flows. The points used in treatments are carefully chosen by the TCM practitioner to disperse any blockages and to bring the patient's Qi into balance.

Moxibustion is the process whereby a dried herb is burnt, either directly on the skin or indirectly above the skin over specific acupuncture points to warm the Qi and Blood in the channels. Moxibustion is most commonly used when there is a requirement to expel Cold and Dampness from the body.

The Yin / Yang symbol is ancient. It first appeared in Chinese historical documents nearly three thousand years ago. The diagram which most people are familiar with as the Yin / Yang symbol is also known as the Tai Chi symbol.

The original meaning and characteristics of these two basic qualities come from: 1) the dark (Yin) shady side of a mountain, 2) the light (Yang) sunlit side of a mountain. In place of the mountain it is considered that a person is standing and facing away from the sun. Therefore the front of the body is relatively Yin and the back of the body is relatively Yang.

"The One Begets the Two". Chinese philosophers have over a period of several hundred years differentiated the chi of the Universe into two forces, Yin and Yang. The quality of Yang was more rarefied, immaterial and vaster; it therefore floated upwards to form the Heavens. Yin was more condensed and material, it sank down and created Earth. As a theory Yin / Yang is a view of the Universe based upon centuries of experience and observation by the Chinese people.

It should be noted that it is only a theory. However, it is an all encompassing, yet flexible, theory and at the same time a simple tool that, once learnt, can be used to explain any number of phenomena. Its qualities are not exclusive, but complementary and relative. Life is not black and white, but a scale of colours ranging from one end of the spectrum to the other and always changing.

The Yin / Yang Symbol

1. The circle symbolizes the wholeness and infinity of chi. There is no beginning nor ending, and pervades through everything. This outer circle is the cosmos that contains the Yang (light) and the Yin (dark).

2. The dividing line between the two sectors is a curved one. This denotes movement and a constant flowing of Yin into Yang and Yang into Yin. It signifies the eternal motion of the combined elements.

3. Within the largest portion (when it has peaked and grown as big as it possibly can) of each colour there is a dot of the opposing colour. This can be considered as a small seed. Therefore we see that there is a small black dot (seed) in the white section and a small white dot (seed) in the black section. Everything contains the seed of its opposite within it. This is symbolic that all things contain both Yin and Yang.

4.　The two colours are in equal proportion, equally balanced. When there is more of one aspect, then there is less of the other.

The relationship of Yin to Yang

Although yin and yang may appear to be opposites, they only exist by virtue of each other. Things are yin or yang only in relation to other things. i.e. dark and light; night and day; earth and heaven; front and back; down and up; cold and hot. It must be understood that one thing can be Yin to another and Yang in relation to a third, i.e. earth is Yin in relation to heaven; heaven is Yang in relation to earth; earth is Yin in relation to the sun (which is hotter) earth is Yang in relation to the moon (which is cooler) Or: tepid is Yin in relation to hot; fiery hot is Yang in relation to hot; icy is Yin in relation to cold; moderately cold is Yang in relation to cold.

CHAPTER 4:   I'LL TRY ANYTHING ONCE

In late September 2005, as part of my undaunting quest to overcome the effects of my illness, I began a series of strategies that included acupuncture therapy and Chinese medicine twice daily. Let me tell you what an adventure that was.

I was gradually being introduced to the Chinese culture and Eastern medicine through some acquaintances I had met in my Taoist Tai Chi classes. After all, as my wife and I often tell ourselves and others, 2.5 billion Chinese can't be far off the mark (suggesting that after 2,000 years, the Chinese must have developed some medicinal expertise)! Through a woman we had met in one of the local Tai Chi classes that we participate in regularly, we were referred to an elderly Chinese gentleman who administered authentic 'deep' acupuncture. This form of acupuncture is the type that is most recognized and recommended for treatment of varying serious and complex illnesses and/or conditions. We had to undergo quite an ordeal to access this man and his skills. He had studied acupuncture in China and was the head acupuncturist in one of the largest hospitals in China. At the time we started seeing him, he had over 46 years' experience. He is a quiet-spoken man, very bright and pleasant-looking but COULDN'T SPEAK MUCH ENGLISH. He was, however, eventually able to express his intentions and requirements, instructing me reasonably well. The language problem, however, did make it quite difficult to understand what he was trying to do as he applied his craft. Don't get me wrong, he was an amazing man and knew what he was doing.

At each session of acupuncture treatment that he gave me, he instilled within me the greatest confidence and always made me feel the calmest you could imagine and made any and all discomfort or pain I was feeling at the time go away.

I find acupuncture to be an unreal experience. The doctor was quite quick and deliberate in his application of the needles. It was quite painless and actually the entire process was relaxing. The doctor lived in a tiny one bedroom apartment and treated me in his front room. He had me lie down on my side on a couch covered with a clean sheet. Usually, his wife was working in the adjoining kitchen and occasionally babysitting their granddaughter while their daughter worked.

As I lay on the couch, I began to doze off and, other than the occasional pleasantry with the doctor, I faded into a calm half-sleep, similar to the snooze one would have while getting a shampoo and haircut or even while having your teeth cleaned during a visit to the dentist.

The first thing the doctor did was take my pulse on both of my wrists and then he examined my tongue. On each visit he felt that my tongue, fortunately, was pink and healthy, indicating he could proceed with the treatment. Before commencing an acupuncture session, he always looked at my hand and pulled at and kneaded my knuckles and tendons, forming my hand in its intended natural position. He pressed down on my swollen and hardened knuckles until my fingers had straightened reasonably. They obviously indicated that more exercise and strengthening would be beneficial. Previously, a physiotherapist had suggested that exercises with a ball might cause my hand to close and tighten further, as opposed to opening. It seems to me that there is no consensus on what is the most desirable way of straightening my fingers. All I know is that I am determined to be able to play guitar again and I have let my doctor and my physiotherapists know that this is my goal. Overall, I believe I had more than twenty visits to this acupuncturist.

Another thing he was strong on was the use of Chinese medicine. He gave us a pre-bagged package of four bags of Chinese medicine, each bag good for three doses or cups of tea. Each bag contained an assortment of plant extracts, tree bark, etc. which Hélène put in a special clay pot and covered with three cups of water. She then brought this concoction to a boil, turned the burner down and then let it simmer until the liquid had been reduced to one cup. I then drank this after I had let it cool down a bit. It was quite vile and nasty tasting, but I was willing to try anything! The doctor maintained it would help my kidneys and my dizziness. My family physician, who coincidentally is also Chinese, maintained that this medicine would take a while to be effective because it is taken in such a small dose.

The acupuncture itself will improve my circulation and, as a result, my mobility. I certainly find it to be very helpful in reducing my pain and discomfort.

Acupuncture is the insertion of hair-like needles into the skin through pressure points which can be found on some 14 major meridians (energy pathways). Each meridian links to a specific organ or organ system.

The theory of acupuncture recognizes that the disharmony of energy in the body creates chronic illnesses while blockage of energy creates pain and weakens the immune system.

Acupuncture directly rebalances the energy by needles and therefore reinstalls health.

The theory of acupuncture coincides with the theory of energy physics by Dr. Albert Einstein – NO ENERGY, NO GROWTH, a theory that explains the phenomenon of electricity or energy while Murphy's Law fails to do so.

Acupuncture has no side effects whatsoever if applied correctly. The use of acupuncture for patients who have difficulty taking prescription drugs may help to reduce or eliminate the intake of such. Furthermore, the effect of acupuncture is usually long lasting!

All chronic situations and pains such as migraine, joint pains, arthritis, sciatica, menstrual pain, high blood pressure, high cholesterol, diabetes, sexual dysfunction, infertility, skin problems, anxiety, overweight and smoking to name a few, can be treated by acupuncture. While acupuncture is well known for its pain management abilities, face lifting is also gaining in popularity due to the natural approach!

For pain management, results can likely be expected in just one session. Other chronic situations usually take longer depending on each individual's health situation. Someone considering acupuncture should call his/her intended practitioner for a free consultation.

Most health insurance plans now cover acupuncture treatments. Some may require a doctor's recommendation.

So, after checking me over, the doctor would go to his desk drawer and take out six or seven cello-sealed needles and place them one at a time at the appropriate points. Occasionally, another client would arrive and sometimes the doctor would excuse himself while he took care of the other client with a quick application of acupuncture. These clients were mostly Chinese and weren't quite as afflicted as I am and therefore didn't need the same attention as me.

The doctor usually started the process by inserting the first needle just below my shoulder, which I understand is intended to simply relax me. Then, he inserted a needle just below my elbow on my forearm, followed by a third one lower down on my forearm, just above my wrist. He then inserted four strategically-placed needles in my lower leg. The needles were left in place for approximately 30 minutes, during which time I was told not to move. During that time, I usually had the most wonderful power snooze!

Just so you realize, as an outcome of my stroke, I often feel the most miserable pain and discomfort in my face, neck, toes, fingers and hand (thalamic pain). After a few moments of the actual application of the acupuncture needles, which he inserts in my left foot, leg, ankle, knee, hand, fingers and face, I often reflected on just how good I felt and how much at peace my body was once more. Hélène and I would often reflect on the mysticism of the VooDoo I was undergoing. Therefore, we faithfully made the long trip down the Don Valley Parkway downtown to Chinatown twice a week and visited the doctor to receive his wonderful acupuncture treatment. It always made me feel so relieved and relaxed. I would sleep solidly for half an hour or more and all my aches and pains would litterally disappear.

As incredibly intelligent and knowledgable as this man was, he unfortunately spoke only a few words of English and we could barely communicate. As he was unable to explain what he was doing to me, it was nothing more than a relationship of trust and few words.

So, one day, on or about the 1st of February, 2006, we decided to see if we could find an alternative acupuncturist who was a little closer to home. We were feeling a little overwhelmed with our entire situation. The treatments were costly, the travel to see the doctor downtown was too time-consuming and parking was expensive and always hard to find. Hélène scanned the local Yellow Pages and lo-and-behold! BINGO! She came across an acupuncturist right here in town, actually just a few blocks from our home. We were so pleased. Our quality of life had just improved significantly. Erik is Chinese also, speaks fluent English and French and explains everything he does for me clearly. He is a certified practitioner and after my first series of treatments with him, I am more than a little impressed. His treatment room is professionally appointed. It is finished and decorated with beige 2'x2' acoustic tile equipped with subdued lighting with appropriately positioned and dimmer-controlled spot-lights. He has a desk and file cabinet in one corner of his office, with the treatment bed parallel and against the far wall, opposite the entrance door. A small foot stool is placed beside the treatment bed to assist patients, the likes of me, to get up and onto the gurney-style bed. Erik prefers to have his FM radio softly playing sometimes country or even 60's or classic rock music in the background. The aura of the room is relaxing and comforting as he proceeds to insert as many as fifteen or more needles gently and painlessly into my face, head, neck, hands, arms, legs, feet and stomach. The result is total relaxation and soon this human pincushion is sound asleep, oblivious to the outside world and totally trusting in the process. Toward the end of a typical one hour treatment, I begin to slowly and gently wake up.

Erik and I chatted recently about the approach he is taking in administering my herbal medicine and acupuncture treatments, which is to:

1. decrease liver yang (tension);
2. increase kidney yin;
3. increase and unblock energy circulation, thereby bringing clarity to the mind.

Erik also recently gave me a list of the ingredients in the herbal (Chinese) medicine I am currently taking twice a day. These include Cimicifugae Rhizoma, Rehmannia, Achyranthes, Pueraria root, Licorice, Angelicae Sinensis Radix, Peony (red) Ligusticum and Lermbricus. We also chatted about his background and some of his origins. I learned that he actually speaks Chui Chau and not any one of the usual Standard Mandarin or Cantonese dialects. About one-fifth of the people in the world speak some form of Chinese as their native language, making it the language with the most native speakers.

In general, all varieties of Chinese are tonal and analytic. However, Chinese is also distinguished for a high level of internal diversity. Regional variation between different dialects is comparable to the Romance language family; many variants of spoken Chinese are different enough to be mutually incomprehensible. There are between six and twelve main regional groups, depending on classification scheme, of which the most populous are Mandarin, Wu, and Cantonese, in that order.

The identification of the varieties of Chinese as "languages" or "dialects" is controversial. The standardized form of spoken Chinese is based on the Beijing dialect, a member of the Mandarin group. Standard Mandarin is the official language of the People's Republic of China as well as one of four official languages of Singapore, together with English, Malay, and Tamil. Chinese (Standard Mandarin) is one of the six official languages of the United Nations, along with English, Arabic, French, Russian, and Spanish. Spoken in the form of Standard Cantonese, Chinese, together with English, is one of the official languages of Hong Kong and of Macau, together with Portuguese.

Chinese linguists have recently distinguished three more groups from the traditional seven:

1. Jin, from Mandarin
2. Hui, from Wu
3. Ping, partly from Cantonese

There are also many smaller groups that are not yet classified, such as: Danzhou dialect, spoken in Danzhou, on Hainan Island; Xianghua, not to be confused with Xiang, spoken in Western Hunan; and Shaozhou Tuhua, spoken in northern Guangdong. The Dungan language, spoken in Central Asia, is very closely related to Mandarin. However, it is not generally considered "Chinese" because it is written in Cyrillic and spoken by people outside China who are not considered Chinese in any sense.

In general, the above languages (dialect groups) do not have sharp boundaries. As with many areas that were linguistically diverse for a long time, it is not always clear how the speeches of various parts of China should be classified. The Ethnologue lists a total of 14, but the number varies between seven and seventeen depending on the classification scheme being followed. In any case, some dialects belonging to the same group may be mutually unintelligible, while other dialects split up among several groups may in fact share many similarities due to geographical proximity.

On the Western Front

I am also occasionally working out at Variety Village, a health and wellness centre that is fortunately only about 25 minutes from our home, in East Scarborough. Variety Clubs International now has over 10,000 members in 60 clubs in 14 countries. Variety International, the 'Children's Charity' is dedicated to improving the lives of children throughout the world. The International President of Variety International is Ory Slonin. This centre has a unique Sports Training and Fitness Centre. Variety – The Children's Charity has been recognized as a world leader in offering progressive state-of-the-art programming and services for children and adults of all abilities. The Village has been providing both a facility to enjoy and a place of hope and encouragement for individuals with special needs for close to 25 years. Approximately 3,000 children and youth with special needs depend on Variety Village for safe, healthy sports programming each week.

Variety Village provides essential sport and fitness programs using a proven integrated model that helps individuals of all abilities develop a greater sense of independence, self-worth, confidence and well-being. With a focus on ability, rather than disability, Variety Village has a reputation for making a real difference in the lives of its members.

Variety Village allows its members to see that they have the ability to do things they thought they could never do. By seeking solutions, rather than focusing on problems, Variety sends everyone a strong message: There is always a way – it simply takes imagination and determination.

I use some of their specialized equipment, specifically the Moto-Med, a machine that enables smooth and safe, bicycle type motion combined with motor aided peddling and monitored and bio-feedback assisted exercise. The Reck MOTO-med is an electrically driven exerciser which provides full cycling exercise without any effort on your part. It is controllable for speed and direction of motion by a hand held remote control. It instantly detects any muscle spasm and responds by stopping and reversing very slowly. It can also be used without the motor for active exercise.

Regular exercise on the MOTO-med will:
- Reduce muscle spasm
- Improve muscle tone
- Improve joint flexibility
- Improve blood circulation
- Stimulate metabolism

While surfing the internet one day about two years ago, in search of solutions to my mobility issues, I came across a device called the NeuroMove. This high-tech equipment was developed to combine the beneficial effects of both biofeedback and muscle stimulation in helping someone who has had a stroke regain some muscle control of their affected limbs.

Electrodes are attached to the muscles through sticky pads and connected to the machine. The electrodes pick up electrical signals which the brain sends to the muscle when it intends to move and rewards the patient with a movement that visually contracts the muscle. The NeuroMove then prompts the patient to relax, the effect of which is reduced tone and an additional voluntary control.

While the results will vary from patient to patient, I found this device to be quite helpful in stimulating my left hand to open voluntarily and naturally. I also found good results when using the NeuroMove on my left foot to encourage dorsiflexion.

I always ended each session on a positive note, feeling encouraged and progressively alive.

CHAPTER 5:   NOT A QUITTER

In June, 2004, about 15 months after I had my first stroke, I began to play wheelchair tennis with an organization called the Ontario Wheelchair Sports Association. They offer a program called *"Bridging the Gap"* and the Coordinator of the program (at that time) was a woman named Leigh.

At the time, Hélène and I had been talking to someone who had told us about wheelchair tennis. He had given us a magazine article about Frank Peter Jr, who is one of the foremost wheelchair tennis players in Canada. The article mentioned that the Canadian National Wheelchair Tennis Championships were coming up that month in Stoney Creek, Ontario. Neither Hélène nor I had ever heard of, let alone seen, wheelchair tennis and we were fascinated and eager to find out what it was all about.

So, on a beautiful Saturday in June, off we went to Stoney Creek. After watching these people spin and reach and hustle for the tennis balls, I was hooked! Leigh was there and she introduced us to several other players, as well as to a gentleman named Richard who kindly offered to give me some one-on-one coaching during the clinic that was to be held a couple of days later. We drove back to Stoney Creek on Monday and I spent most of the day working with Richard, learning how to adapt my strokes to my new situation. It was truly amazing.

Shortly afterwards, Leigh emailed an invitation to us to attend wheelchair tennis sessions at a Tennis Centre not too far from our home. Initially, we would drive up there every Thursday night and play outdoors for a couple of hours. This went on until the colder weather hit and court time was no longer available.

Unfortunately, I had difficulty finding someone to play with during the winter months, so I was forced to put my game "on the back burner", so to speak.

Then, after enquiring several times about playing again, I discovered that a group was starting up indoors at the same location on Monday nights this time. We are usually 5 or 6 players and we play for two hours every week. Unlike the others, I have the added challenge of having to play in my powered wheelchair, while everyone else plays in a sports wheelchair. My left side paralysis makes it impossible for me to propel a manual chair with both hands. Controlling my chair while holding my tennis racquet and a tennis ball is quite a challenge, but I persist and I do enjoy it tremendously!

As well, I found it particularly difficult to play with individuals who happen to be also confined to wheelchairs, but who still have their upper body strength and ability. You see, these athletes are usually accident victims who have spinal cord injuries and therefore no longer have use of their legs or lower body. Therefore, they can use both arms to toss and serve a tennis ball. However, having suffered a stroke and the resultant brain damage that affected my left side, I cannot propel a wheelchair or toss and reasonably serve a ball. I therefore find my ability in the game to be considerably weaker competitively than most other wheelchair tennis athletes. So, for the time being, I have decided to avoid the whole aspect of playing wheelchair tennis. It is too frustrating and disappointing. I am hoping, however, to attempt to organize some wheelchair tennis for similarly afflicted individuals who have restrictions on one side of their body, as opposed to problems with the lower half of their bodies.

CHAPTER 6: A NEW LIFE... FORE!

Today, Tuesday, July 26, 2005, has been an incredible start to a new chapter in the development of the continuation of my new life. Before I had my strokes, I played tennis competitively and dabbled at golf, playing 18 holes maybe five or six times a year, only ever breaking 100 once or twice. Unfortunately, my unyielding power usually resulted in the ugliest drive and most incredible slices into the woods! You can just imagine how much I miss that independence, including the invaluable sportsmanship and competitiveness.

Well, today was a monumental day. I met a couple of amazing golf pros who were incredibly supportive and keen to ensure I got on the right track by fitting me with the appropriate length clubs for use from my power wheelchair, thus making it possible for me to have the game of golf back in my life. Jeff Swain is the professional club fitter at Angus Glen Golf Club. He evaluated my current clubs and determined what he thought would be the best length for me to play effectively, given the fact that I will be playing sitting in my wheelchair. He suggested an oversized driver and said that he thought he had some heads at home with which he could supply me, so all I would have to buy would be the shafts.

After hitting a few balls and getting some tips on position, etc., Jeff introduced Hélène and me to the Assistant Golf Pro, Paul Bussiere. Hélène expressed interest in taking golf lessons so that she and I can enjoy the game together. She and Paul will set up a time that works for both of them so that she can be properly introduced to the game.

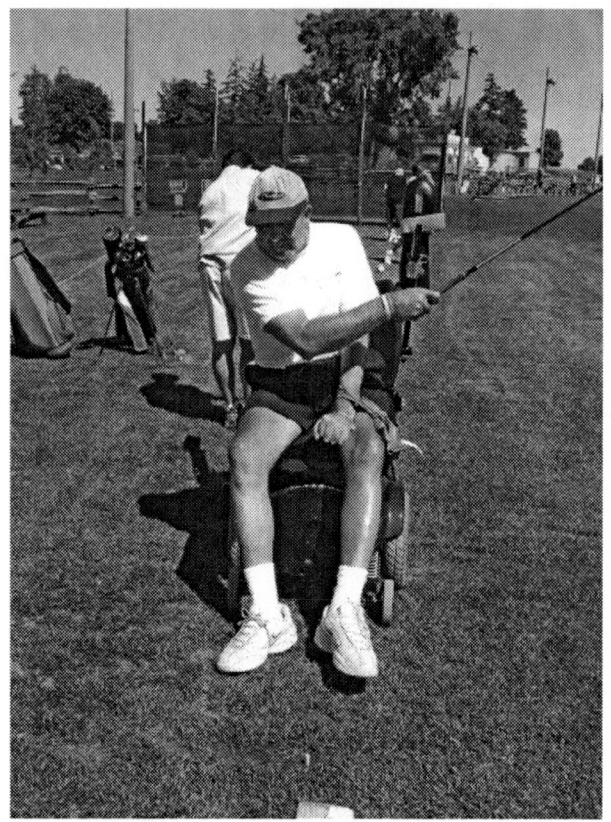

Wheelchair golf, August 2005

As we drove home, I looked over lovingly at Hélène and told her gently "Thank you for coming out here with me today, hon" and she replied caringly and with her cute little smile, "No problem, babe. I enjoyed it. I see that you did too!" observing the happy gaze in my eyes, having taken the first critical steps to reestablishing one of the passions of my former life since my new disability. I still am not quite certain that this particular activity can actually fit into our already overwhelming schedule, particularly at this time while we are busily trying to finish this book. We'll see. You know me. I'll give it a damn good try.

CHAPTER 7: MY RECOVERY HOBBY: AND HERE THEY ARE... THE BEATLES

When I was just about 10 years old, I became a huge Beatles fan. By the time I was 14, my Dad had purchased an electric guitar for me. My friends and I were playing in bands by the time I was 16 and I learned a lot about playing guitar from them. I still remember a comment Gordie made while we were jamming together one day. He said "Holy frig, can this guy ever play lead!" I began my wonderful collection of Beatles' albums and it had become very easy to buy me Christmas and birthday gifts. In fact, I was such a huge Beatles fan that my Mom, being British, took me to see the Beatles at the Montreal Forum on September 8, 1964. I was then only 11. Beatles music continued to mean so much to me that I was playing it in my latest band right up until four days before my stroke and I was by then, of course, a graceful and learned "49 years old"!

One day way back then, my Mom was speaking to her sister, my dear Auntie Stella, who lives overseas. It was arranged that Auntie Stella would subscribe to the Beatles Monthly Fan Club Book and would send me the latest issue each month. I was thrilled at this marvelous collection at the time and somehow, while growing up and even with my typical adolescent interests and activities, I managed to take great care of these books and, even today, I still have a significant portion of a cherished nearly complete collection in near mint condition.

Now, having had a major stroke at 49 years of age and while in the process of writing about my life and near fatal illness, I have renewed my fascination with this collection. Never having for a moment lost my appreciation of the Fab Four, I was surfing the internet one day recently and came across a sale on eBay, which listed for auction a number of volumes of Beatles Monthly Books. I pulled out my collection and did a thorough inventory, taking note of the issues I had never actually owned in the first place, because they were from the beginning of the series. It would appear that it was only in December of 1963 that I actually started receiving these magazines regularly. I quickly determined that I was missing issues 1, 2, 3, 5 and 8 or those from August, September, October and December, 1963 as well as March of 1964. I had all the others, still in mint condition, up to #48. For some reason, I had #48 -July, 1967 and was missing #49 - August, 1967. I simply concluded that perhaps Johnny Dean, the series' editor, had probably ceased publication of the books beyond #49. So I keenly started to peruse the auctions and quickly discovered that there were several Beatles Monthly Books available. Over the next four or five weeks, Hélène and I successfully negotiated and outbid other Beatles fans to eventually attain all of the issues I had been missing in between. I was delighted to complete what I considered to be a very special and invaluable collection of famous memorabilia that my dear Auntie Stella had initiated for me over 40 years ago. I now had every issue from #1 to #50, in good condition at that.

I must tell you though, how both pleased but shocked I was when I learned, upon investigating, that the series had actually not ended at #50. I continued to browse eBay and discovered that some vendors were actually selling issues beyond #50! I successfully bid on and won issues for the years 1991 and 1996. I have been continuing my quest. Upon a little more investigation with one of the eBay Beatles Book vendors, I learned that these books had continued into the year 2001 for 38 more years or 456 more issues!

So, once more, it seems as though I am missing "a few" issues; however, I am still interested in continuing and completing this wonderful set and will pursue my quest for missing issues until I am satisfied that my collection is as complete as reasonably possible. It is sure to be invaluable some day.

CHAPTER 8:   SUPPORT GROUPS

About a year and a half or so after my discharge from Bridgepoint Health, Hélène and I discovered a stroke survivors' support group which met once a week in our area. Anyone who has been through this kind of trauma can certainly benefit from other people's experience and encouragement.

We attended these meetings every Tuesday afternoon and always felt very welcome and very much a part of the group, right from Day One. We would invite guest speakers every two weeks or so and would do some kind of activity on the other Tuesdays. Our regular routine always included an exercise program, a business meeting, some discussion on a variety of outside activities that members of the group might or might not wish to participate in and, of course, coffee, tea and cookies!

The meetings were held in a local church and were somewhat informal, although the business portion of the meeting was more structured.

Unfortunately, after about a year of attending and enjoying these meetings, I began acupuncture treatments which, because of the doctor's busy schedule, could only happen at the same time as the support group meetings. I had no choice but to quit the group. I did, however, appreciate the encouragement and support all these wonderful people gave me during my time with them and I wish them all well.

As my journey continues I remain uncertain of what the outcome of my recovery will be. True, I have made what some are calling "outstanding progress", considering I was once practically comatose and indefinitely confined to a hospital bed. I am now limited to using a wheelchair as my legs. However, I have taught myself to hit golf balls and to play tennis and since last year (2005), I have learned to enter the pool with assistance usually from my lovely and ever-present wife and I am able to swim a number of lengths of our 16 x 32' pool as soon as I get in the heated 95 degree F water. I cannot express emphatically enough how glorious it feels to finally be in the water again, stretching and kicking and reaching forward with each stroke, albeit with only one good arm. Even though my left side is supposedly paralyzed, I am fortunately able to kick with my stiff left leg because my hip seems to be strong and does work. I suppose it is more a part of my central physical makeup and body structure than just part of my paralyzed left side. The result, therefore, is a near perfect typical swim-kick. A near miracle, I'd say.

So now, three and a half years later, I am walking, albeit with a side walker. Today I was again in our pool with Hélène and was swimming lengths without my life jacket which I usually always had to wear. This summer, I started to swim without it for the first time since my stroke. Last year, my determination and perseverance saw me do intentional belly flops, from the top step, to immediately enter the four foot deep pool and promptly swim ten to fifteen lengths at a time. This year, when I first got into the pool at the beginning of the summer, I immediately swam a few lengths but as I always found getting into the life jacket a bit of a hassle and quite simply an annoying, uncomfortable, unwelcome extra step, I decided to attempt my laps without it. In my previous life, I was a reasonably proficient and capable swimmer. Getting into the water now, even in my new, crippled state, I am still confident. Being a non-smoker, I have good, strong lungs and am extremely relaxed in the water. I stand upright in the weightless buoyancy then, falling forward, I push off, submerge my head, splashing face first then launch myself into the first of ten or fifteen consecutive lengths. I can still sustain a good breath and easily swim two laps without needing to come up for a breath of air. Swimming every day has given me back some independence, which is a salvation for me. I enjoy the stretch, the relaxing and the exercise it provides me with so much. Hélène tells me over and over again how proud of me she is.

Another recent marvelous discovery we have made has been HIAD (The Head Injury Association of Durham Region). This is an organization dedicated to assisting people who have suffered any one of a range of different brain injuries.

I attended my first session at their facility in Durham two or three weeks ago and again last Thursday. A discussion group meets every Thursday afternoon, giving a number of us who are similarly afflicted an opportunity to talk about any of a broad range of issues or problems we are encountering or experiencing. These are issues that people who have had traumatic head injuries or who have experienced a stroke want and need to discuss with others who are in the same situation. We share our experiences and problems and try to make our world and our environment a better place in which to live.

I refer to the following quote from Marlies, one of a number of good Taoist Tai Chi friends of mine: "Illness and loss change life but don't make it less worth living." It is so typical of her. She is such an inspiration. I shall never forget her. She made such a difference to me whenever we worked together on my recovery and I look forward to our next meeting on Awareness Day.

I discovered a chat group for stroke survivors on the internet in March, 2005, after thinking for the longest time that it would be helpful to be able to talk and listen to other stroke survivors about their experiences, problems and challenges. I am thrilled to have discovered this group and heartily recommend exploring it to anyone who is in my situation and indeed for anyone who is simply interested in finding out more about stroke and its effects and challenges, whether they are caregivers, family or just good friends.

You can find this and other similar chat groups through your internet search engine.

Work like you don't need the money,
Love like you've never been hurt,
And dance as if no one was watching.

SECTION NINE – A FEW THINGS YOU SHOULD KNOW

CHAPTER 1: HIGH BLOOD PRESSURE AND WHAT IT CAN DO TO YOU

High blood pressure is just as common in younger men as it is in their older counterparts and should be taken just as seriously by both age groups. You're under 35 and feel fine, yet the doctor says your blood pressure is high and you'd better come back to have it checked again. Being a red-blooded male, you figure five years will be soon enough. After all, isn't high blood pressure an old man's disease?

Young men are less likely than older men to believe they have hypertension and less likely to go back to the doctor. Often these are patients whose blood pressure would respond positively to weight management and other lifestyle changes, but they are less likely to seek treatment.

Untreated hypertension damages the heart and other organs and can lead to life-threatening conditions that include heart disease, stroke, and kidney disease. It is called "the silent killer" because symptoms generally appear only after the disease has caused damage to vital organs. Timely treatment can truly prolong life.

If your blood pressure is 120/80, 120 represents systolic pressure or the pressure of blood against artery walls when the heart beats; 80 represents diastolic pressure or the pressure between beats.

Normal	Less than 120/80
Pre-hypertension	120-139/80-89

Hypertension	140/90 (130/80 for patients with diabetes or chronic kidney disease)
Stage 2 hypertension	160/100

My blood pressure, just before I had my strokes, was floating between 160/90 and 180/90. My blood pressure now, since I am on a strictly monitored and carefully prescribed program, is safely between 110/78 and 120/80.

Hypertension, or high blood pressure, exists when either the systolic measurement is 140 or higher or the diastolic measurement is 90 or higher. However, in the majority of people, controlling systolic hypertension is a more important heart disease risk factor than diastolic blood pressure, except in young people under the age of 50.

There are two types of hypertension: essential, which accounts for 90% to 95% of cases, and secondary. The cause of essential hypertension is unknown, although lifestyle factors such as obesity, sedentary lifestyle, and excessive alcohol or salt intake contribute to the condition. The cause of secondary hypertension may be kidney disease; hormonal imbalance; or drugs, including cocaine or alcohol.

Because blood pressure increases with age, most people will become hypertensive if they live long enough. According to the JNC 7, half the adult population is pre-hypertensive or hypertensive. The JNC 7 is the seventh report of the Joint National Committee on Prevention, Detection, Evaluation and Treatment of High Blood Pressure. Hypertension is usually diagnosed upon finding blood pressure of 140/90 mmHg or above, measured on both arms. Because blood pressure readings in many individuals are highly variable, especially in the office setting, the diagnosis of hypertension should be made only after noting a mean elevation on two or more readings during two or more office visits, unless the elevations are severe or associated with compelling indications such as diabetes mellitus, chronic kidney disease, heart failure, post-myocardial infarction, stroke, or high coronary disease risk. Recently, the JNC 7 has defined blood pressure of 120/80 mmHg to 139/89 mmHg as "prehypertension." Prehypertension is not a disease category; rather, it is a designation chosen to identify individuals at high risk of developing hypertension.

CHAPTER 2: STROKE, COMPLEX CENTRAL PAIN SYNDROME AND THALAMIC PAIN SYNDROME

A stroke, or cerebrovascular accident (CVA), occurs when the blood supply to a part of the brain is suddenly interrupted. Stroke is classified by its cause into two main types: *ischemic* and *hemorrhagic*. In an ischemic stroke, which accounts for approximately 90% of strokes, a blood vessel becomes occluded and the blood supply to part of the brain is totally or partially blocked. Ischemia, a reduction of blood flow, most commonly due to occlusion (obstruction) of a blood vessel, leads to a potentially deadly ischemic cascade in brain tissue.

A hemorrhagic stroke, or intracranial hemorrhage, occurs in about 10% of strokes, when a blood vessel or cerebral aneurysm in the brain bursts, spilling blood into the spaces surrounding the brain cells. The mortality and long-term morbidity prognosis is generally worse for hemorrhagic strokes than for ischemic strokes. A small proportion of strokes are watershed strokes caused by hypoperfusion, usually due to hypotension or other vascular problems including vasculitis.

Stroke, the third leading cause of death and the leading cause of adult disability in the US, Canada and industrialized European nations, is a medical emergency. It generally presents itself to the victim with loss of function in the area of the body controlled by the affected part of the brain, such as hemiplegia, loss of speech or vision, impaired swallowing reflex or altered sensation. The immediate and long-term results lead to varying degrees of morbidity and even mortality. To illustrate the seriousness of a stroke, the term *brain attack* has become increasingly popular in recent years, in relation to the established term *heart attack*, which is used for myocardial infarctions.

There are a couple of known pain syndromes associated with stroke:

Sinus headaches are a pain. Backaches, toothaches, sprains, strains all cause pain of some kind and at some level. We have all experienced some pain at one time or another in our lives. Some people swear by acetaminophen, others Ibuprofen, NSAIDS of different forms, all the way up to the big guns of Narcotics. Most of the pains mentioned previously go away at some point.

But for many of us, there is another pain, one with various names, that stays with us almost always. We call it Central Pain Syndrome, CPS for short.

CPS is also known as Thalamic Pain Syndrome, Dejerine-Roussy Syndrome, Posterior Thalamic Syndrome, Retrolenticular Syndrome, Central Post-Stroke Syndrome and is often found under Neuropathic Pain. You may have heard it referred to by any of these names, or perhaps even something else.

Central Pain Syndrome is a neurological condition, meaning it stays with us, can affect us all differently, in different places on our bodies and at different levels of pain. It is also extremely difficult to diagnose, sometimes sending the patient to many doctors to find one that believes them and/or has even heard of and dealt with and treated this savage pain.

Caused by damage to the central nervous system by stroke, it also includes thalamus; brainstem; spinal cord injury; MS; reaction to medications; TBI injuries; and other conditions.

It can be a steady, sometimes deep burning, aching, cutting, tearing sensation. CPS may be mixed with sudden, excruciating shots of pain. It is often mixed with other distracting sensations like cold, tingling, a "pins and needles" effect, a ballooning sensation, throbbing, and the feeling of a dental probe on a raw nerve.

Intense skin reactions can accompany these symptoms, such as burning, stretching, tightness, itching or a crawling feeling that can be irritated by any light touch, sometimes just the feel of cloth on skin, which can make dressing an ordeal. Sometimes the touch of a loved one or family member, in fun or love, may often be a way to overwhelm the brain with the pain from CPS.

Sometimes the hands and feet are affected with a numbness that is painful and does not offer any relief, only adding to the pain. It is often aggravated by temperature changes, particularly cold.

It can take months, even years, after a stroke to make its appearance, well after the patient thinks they are well on the road to recovery. CPS can often cause depression, anxiety, anger and frustration.

In some cases, when a person rates the pain as a 9 or 10 on a pain scale and there seems to be no relief in sight, no hope or understanding with support, they may even come to feel that suicide is the only way out. In that way Central Pain Syndrome can be a life threatening condition.

The following triggers have been identified which can start or increase one's sensations and pain levels: Movement, daily activity, ROM exercising, exposure to sun, cold, breezes, AC, barometer changes, weather (hot and cold, rain, snow), real pain or swelling, stress, anger, depression. touches of another person, blankets, clothes, splints, tiredness, sudden movements such as yawning and other reflexive involuntary movements like sneezing, being startled, fear, vibrations such as when riding in a car.

Complex central pain syndrome is sometimes called *Thalamic Pain*, since it is believed to originate as a result of stroke damage to the thalamic gland which is situated above the brainstem. The thalamus affects our feelings of hot and cold.

Regardless of the name, the pain is neurological in origin and affects a number of stroke victims. The pain varies from mild to quite severe. It usually does not appear until quite some time (e.g. a year) after the stroke. Complex central pain syndrome, however, is not exclusive to stroke victims.

Thalamic pain syndrome is characterized by chronic pain occurring on the same side of the body that is affected by the stroke, opposite the side of the brain on which the stroke occurred.

Deep beneath the surface of each of the two globe-like halves of the brain is a group of berry and nut-sized clusters of brain cells collectively known as the *basal ganglia*. One of the more central of these clusters is called the Thalamus. The Thalamus acts as a central processing center for sensory information streaming toward the brain from the rest of the body. Sensory information such as touch, pressure, heat, cold, and pain travels along nerves from all parts of the body into the spinal cord, where it travels upward along specialized pathways, or tracts, toward the brain. As all of the various sensory tracts enter the brain through the brainstem, they converge upon the Thalamus, which processes and integrates the multitude of sensations and then relays them to appropriate areas of the brain where the information is used or brought into the individual's conscious awareness.

It is important to note that, as the sensory tracts ascend toward the brain, most cross over at some point to the opposite side of the spinal cord or brainstem. For instance, pain sensation from the right hand travels via sensory nerves to enter the right half of the spinal cord, travels a short distance upward in a tract which then crosses over to the left half of the cord to finally deliver the sensory pain message to the left thalamus in the left side of the brain. Thus, a pinprick on the right hand is appreciated mostly in the left half of the brain.

The deep structures of the brain, including the basal ganglia, receive their blood supply from very small, almost hair-thin arteries, called arterioles. Occlusion or blockage of one or more of these arterioles can occur for a variety of reasons, resulting in a small deep stroke often referred to as a "lacunar stroke" or "lacunar infarction." Lacune means "lake" or "hole." Most strokes affecting the thalamus and producing the pain syndrome are of this type. Not all strokes involving the thalamus produce this syndrome, which typically develops weeks or even months after the event. The exact reasons why some thalamic strokes produce it are not well understood.

A small stroke confined mainly to the thalamus will initially produce some loss of sensation on the opposite side of the body. If the stroke damages adjacent brain structures involved in motor function, some degree of paralysis or weakness can occur on the opposite side as well. Typically, the lost functions will partially recover over time. In a few cases, even if the recovery is nearly complete, the pain syndrome begins to develop. It may start as a vague uncomfortable sensation such as stinging of the skin. It may be confined to one limb or to half of the face, or may involve the entire half of the body including face, torso, and limbs. This may progress to true pain, sometimes excruciating in intensity. The character of the pain varies among individuals, and may be described as a burning, hot sensation, shooting or lancing pain, or even feelings of the skin being scratched and torn. The pain is usually unrelenting, present to some degree during all waking hours. In many cases, the normal perception of innocuous sensations may become altered; an individual may perceive light touches, the rub of clothing, or even drafts of air as irritating or painful on the involved side, a condition referred to variously as hypersensitivity, hyperpathia, allodynia, or dysesthesia. The pain syndrome may improve over time, but is often permanent.

The presentation of the thalamic pain syndrome can be confounding to medical practitioners. The usual course is to search for a cause of pain in the limbs, such as arthritis, skin conditions, or pinched nerves. When no physical cause is turned up after exhaustive examinations, the practitioner may characterize the pain as psychological or psychosomatic in nature. The irony is that when a doctor labels the pain as being "all in the patient's head," he is not making an incorrect statement. The pain does indeed originate in the thalamus, inside the brain—it is merely *perceived* by the patient as being located in the involved body parts. Once a diagnosis is made, usually by a physician experienced in the long-term care of stroke survivors, appropriate therapy can be initiated.

Unfortunately, there is no single effective treatment for this disorder. Traditional oral pain medications such as acetaminophen (Tylenol), ibuprofen (Advil, Motrin), naproxen (Naprosyn, Anaprox, Aleve) have limited effect. Combinations of these medications with narcotic analgesics such as codeine or hydrocodone (Vicodyn and others) are somewhat more effective if side effects can be tolerated.

There has been moderate success in recent years with the use of non-traditional or atypical pain medications. These are medicines that were developed to treat other medical conditions such as epileptic seizures or depression, and are now being discovered to have efficacy in the treatment of neurological causes of pain. Amytryptiline (Elavil) and similar antidepressants are used, and early side effects such as dry mouth and sedation can usually be overcome with judicious management. Epileptic seizure drugs are showing even more promise, sometimes with fewer side effects. The most popular of these is gabapentin (Neurontin), and others are slowly coming into use.

The principle followed in application of the non-traditional medications is "Start low and go slow." The drugs are initiated at low doses and gradually increased over weeks to allow the patient to develop tolerance to the side effects. The effect of these medications is not immediate; a patient cannot simply take a tablet during a bout of severe pain and expect the pain to be alleviated. Typically, a patient must have been taking an appropriate dose for a week or weeks for the full beneficial effect to occur. Thus a trial of any one of the medications can take months. If one medication does not work or is not tolerated due to side effects after an appropriate trial, then another medication must be chosen and tried. The finding of an optimum treatment therefore requires patience and perseverance on the part of the patient and the physician. The goal of oral medicinal therapy is not to eliminate the pain, but to make it manageable and tolerable.

Some specialized pain management centers are applying a variety of aggressive procedures for thalamic pain which are too involved to discuss at length here. All have had variable success. These techniques may include implanted pumps to deliver medication into the spinal canal, surgical destruction of areas of the thalamus or basal ganglia near the stroke, or implantation of a wire which delivers low level electrical current to the basal ganglia in an attempt to block pain signals from the thalamus to the rest of the brain.

Although I was fortunate enough to have avoided this type of pain for the first two and a half years following my strokes, I now experience this discomfort on a daily basis. There are times when the pain is so severe I wish I could just go to sleep and never wake up! Sleeping appears to make all my pain go away and allows me to forget everything that has happened to me.

Fortunately, a few months ago my family physician prescribed a new drug that has recently come on the market which seems to be helping. The pharmaceutical name of this drug is "Pregabalin"; the common name is "Lyrica" and I take one or two 75 mg tablets twice a day. It makes most of my pain go away, at least temporarily.

Earlier today, I was feeling particularly bad – a very achy, excruciating pain and pressure in my head and extremities and stiffness in my left arm and leg. My wife just went to the pharmacy to pick up a refill of Lyrica and gave me two when she came home. Within an hour, I was feeling so much better!

Most people have had the experience of having a toothache and going to the dentist to have a filling or even an extraction to fix the problem and make the pain go away. The entire process is, fortunately, usually quite routine and fairly pain and trauma-free. Also, many may experience accidents that cause serious injury, sometimes requiring stitches or some form of reparative procedure. Other accidents may involve broken bones and having to wear a cast to help reset and mend a fracture. Altogether, usually quite painful and hopefully, temporarily inconvenient.

My type of illness, however, involves a myriad of ailments and discomforts. My particular stroke, otherwise referred to as a "brain attack", was the result of two hemorrhagic bleeds compounded by the complications associated with hemophilia. When I experienced the second bleed in my cerebellum, the "pocket" of blood put severe pressure on my brain, shifting it inside my head and causing me to become less and less coherent. In addition, there was evidence of hydrocephalus, or "water on the brain". Once the doctors had examined my CT scan, they quickly realized that I needed to have surgery and fast! They rushed me down to Toronto Western Hospital where, following a four-hour operation that included inserting a shunt in my head to drain the excess fluid from my brain, Hélène and Brian were told by the neurosurgeon that, had I not been rushed in for surgery, I would not have survived the weekend!

Since my initial stroke in February 2003, I was involved in the usual attempts at text-book reparative procedures. Then, soon after my second stroke, I was involved in a carefully monitored rehabilitation process that enabled me to relearn everything from language (I had forgotten the words for many common things) to sitting up on the side of my bed, to eating and swallowing normal food. Once I was discharged and sent home, I was referred to our local community hospital (where I had initially been brought in the ambulance) for outpatient physiotherapy. During my time there, I was taught how to bear weight on my left foot and leg and walk with a side walker. At this point, I still had no control, nor did I have any voluntary movement on my left side. About a year after I had been discharged from the hospital and sent home and had begun the process of rehabilitation, I became aware of this thalamic pain. In fact, I began to endure a continuous, excruciating pain in my fingers and toes and all of the extremities of my left side, including numbness in my lips and face ALL OF THE TIME!

Simply stated, however, I was lucky to be alive!

Please refer to the section; "How I Feel", which actually is a log of the pain and discomfort I had been experiencing over the course of the past few years since the year after my stroke.

CHAPTER 3: COMPLEX REGIONAL PAIN SYNDROME

The second pain syndrome associated with stroke is complex regional pain syndrome. This type of pain may actually occur after an injury to an arm or a leg. In rare cases, the syndrome develops after surgery, a heart attack, a stroke or other medical problem. The pain is often described as a burning feeling and is much worse than expected for the injury. A doctor may also call this condition reflex sympathetic dystrophy or causalgia. The cause of the syndrome is not known.

A doctor will make the diagnosis based on pain symptoms and a physical exam. People with this syndrome still have severe, often burning pain, long after the time when their injuries should have healed. The injured area is often swollen. The color or the temperature and moistness of the skin may change. The skin may be sensitive to a light touch or to changes in temperature.

Usually, no tests are needed to diagnose this condition. A doctor may order x-rays or blood tests to see whether another illness is causing pain.

While medicine can help, no single drug or combination of drugs gives long-lasting relief to patients with this problem. Several medicines are used to treat the pain of complex regional pain syndrome. Medicines that block certain nerves may be prescribed. Sometimes steroids help. Some medicines used for depression and seizures also help this chronic pain. Narcotics and other pain medicines may not control the sting of complex regional pain syndrome.

A doctor may suggest a sympathetic block, an injection of an anesthetic (pain reliever) into certain nerves to block the pain signals. If the injection works, it may be repeated. Physical therapy and psychological counseling are also helpful. However, a treatment that works for one person may not work for another. An individual treatment plan must be made for each person.

With early treatment, you may keep complex regional pain syndrome from getting worse. Sometimes the condition improves. If treatment is started early enough, the symptoms may completely disappear. However, people with more severe symptoms that have lasted for a long time often don't respond to treatment. These people may benefit from a pain management program aimed specifically at dealing with chronic pain.

CHAPTER 4: SLEEP APNEA AND HYPERTENSION

I look normal. I feel far from normal.

It is 2:55 am and I have just suddenly woken after a pretty solid sleep. Most of my sleeps are pretty good actually, falling asleep after watching one of our favourite late shows such as CSI, Crossing Jordan, City Confidential or The First 48. Hélène and I like mostly the same shows except for the odd chick flick that I prefer to fall asleep to. Most nights, we pretty much fall asleep together in each other's arms.

During my stay in the hospital, we discovered that I may have Sleep apnea. Also, I occasionally snore loudly enough that it prevents Hélène from getting to sleep and keeps her from having a solid sleep, most recently keeping her from having even a good sleep altogether.

So, while out shopping at the mall the other day, we stumbled across a pretty complete health food store and discovered some medicines that seemed to fit the bill for a few of our relatively minor but nagging daily and ongoing health problems. One bottle of pills that we discovered was for snoring and Sleep apnea which seemed to advocate that it could control my condition and the symptoms of Sleep apnea which I seem to demonstrate. Well, for a couple of nights after trying the medicine, we were actually finally successful in getting through the night without me snoring and Hélène had a peaceful and complete sleep.

Just to provide some additional background, when I was in the hospital after my stroke, it was determined that I exhibited the classic symptoms of Sleep apnea and the physicians slapped on all this fancy monitoring gear to keep a close eye on my sleeping and breathing.

You see, Sleep apnea is actually a condition that causes you to stop breathing while you may be in the process of sucking in a normal but needed breath. Sometimes this condition is actually regarded as potentially quite serious and must be watched very closely. We were made aware of this issue but, among the thousands of other things on our plate at the time, we had not quite gotten around to looking into this one.

At the time of this writing, in February 2006, we have actually made an appointment for me to have a sleep test at a sleep disorder clinic. The purpose is to look into my snoring and at the same time, identify whether or not I have Sleep apnea and, if so, what they can do about it.

According to the literature we have been given on the subject, Sleep apnea is a disorder in which a person stops breathing during the night, perhaps hundreds of times, usually for periods of ten seconds or longer. In most cases the person is unaware of it, although sometimes they awaken and gasp for breath. It is usually accompanied by snoring. People who have Sleep apnea may not even be aware of the condition, but it inevitably causes daytime sleepiness.

Sleep apnea is generally categorized as obstructive, central, or mixed. A less severe form of obstructed breathing is called Upper Airway Resistance Syndrome (UARS).

Obstructive Sleep Apnea (OSA), the most common form of apnea, occurs when tissues in the upper throat or airway collapse at intervals during sleep, thereby blocking the passage of air. In general, OSA occurs on its way to the lungs as air passes through the nose, mouth, and throat. Under normal conditions, the back of the throat is soft and pliant and tends to collapse inward as a person breathes. Certain muscles, called dilator muscles, work against this to keep the airway open. Interference or abnormalities in this process cause air turbulence.

In some cases, the interference is incomplete (called *obstructive hypopnea*) and causes continuous but slow and shallow breathing. In response, the throat vibrates and makes the sound of snoring. Snoring can occur whether a person breathes through the mouth or the nose. It should be noted that snoring could occur without Sleep apnea.

If the tissues at the back of the throat collapse and become momentarily blocked, *Apnea* occurs. Apnea literally means 'absence of breath'. Apnea decreases the amount of oxygen in the blood, and eventually this lack of oxygen triggers the lungs to suck in air. At this point, the patient may make a gasping or snorting sound but does not usually fully wake up.

Central Sleep Apnea is much less common. It is caused by some problem in the central nervous system, most likely a failure of the brain to signal the airway muscles to breathe. In such cases, oxygen levels drop abruptly and usually the sleeper wakes with a start. Often people with Central Sleep Apnea recall waking up. They generally experience less sleepiness during the day than people with Obstructive Sleep Apnea.

Mixed Apnea is the term used when the two apneas occur together.

Upper Airway Resistance Syndrome (UARS) is a condition in which patients complain about excessive daytime sleepiness and there are symptoms of airway resistance. However, such patients do not necessarily meet the criteria for sleep apnea and they do not show a reduction in oxygen levels in the blood. Unlike apnea, UARS is more likely to occur in women than in men. Treatments are similar to those of sleep apnea. It is not known if UARS has any serious health complications.

In sleep studies, subjects spend about one-third of their time asleep, suggesting that most people need about eight hours of sleep each day. Individual adults differ in the amount of sleep they need to feel well rested, however. Infants may sleep as many as 16 hours a day.

The daily cycle of life, which includes sleeping and waking, is called a *circadian* or "about a day" rhythm, commonly referred to as the biologic clock. Hundreds of bodily functions follow biologic clocks, but sleeping and waking comprise the most prominent circadian rhythm. The sleeping and waking cycle is approximately 24 hours. If confined to windowless apartments, with no clocks or other time cues, sleeping and waking as their bodies dictate, humans typically live on slightly longer than 24-hour cycles. It usually takes the following daily patterns:

Humans are designed for daytime activity and night time rest.

Additionally, there is a natural peak in sleepiness at midday, the traditional siesta time. Also, daily rhythms combine with other factors that may interfere or change individual patterns; the fraction-of-a-second-firing of nerve cells in the brain may be faster or slower in different individuals. The monthly menstrual cycle in women can shift the pattern.

Light signals coming through the eyes reset the circadian cycles each day, so changes in season or various exposures to light and dark may unsettle the pattern. The importance of sunlight as a cue for circadian rhythms is dramatized by the problems experienced by people who are totally blind: they commonly suffer trouble sleeping and other rhythm disruptions. The response to light signals in the brain is an important key factor in sleep: Light signals travel to a tiny cluster of nerves in the hypothalamus in the center of the brain, the body's master clock, which is called the *supra chiasmatic nucleus* or SCN. This nerve cluster takes its name from its location, which is just above (*supra*) the optic chiasm. The optic chiasm is a major junction for nerves transmitting information about light from the eyes.

The approach of dusk each day prompts the SCN to signal the nearby *pineal gland* (named so because it resembles a pinecone) to produce the hormone melatonin.

Melatonin is thought to act as the body's time-setting hormone. The longer a person is in darkness, the longer the duration of melatonin secretion. Secretion can be diminished by staying in bright light. Melatonin also appears to serve as a trigger for the need to sleep.

Sleep consists of two distinct states that alternate in cycles and reflect differing levels of brain nerve cell activity. During a normal night's sleep, one progresses through these stages about five or six times:

Non-Rapid Eye Movement (Non REM) sleep is also termed quiet sleep. Non REM sleep is subdivided into three stages of progression:

Stage 1 (light sleep).
Stage 2 (so-called true sleep).

Stage 3 to 4 (deep "slow-wave" or delta sleep).

With each descending stage, awakening becomes more difficult. It is not known what governs Non REM sleep in the brain. A balance between certain hormones, particularly growth and stress hormones, may be important for 'deep sleep'.

Rapid Eye-Movement (REM) Sleep is termed active sleep and is believed, by some experts, to be regulated by the circadian clock in the hypothalamus. Most vivid dreams occur in REM sleep. REM sleep brain activity is comparable to that in waking but the muscles are virtually paralyzed, possibly preventing people from acting out their dreams. In fact, except for vital organs like lungs and heart, the only muscles not paralyzed during REM sleep are the eye muscles. REM sleep may be critical for learning and for day-to-day mood regulation. When people are sleep-deprived, their brains must work harder than when they are well rested.

The cycle between quiet (Non REM) and active (REM) sleep generally follows this pattern: After about 90 minutes of Non REM sleep, eyes move rapidly behind closed lids, giving rise to REM sleep. As sleep progresses, the Non REM/REM cycle repeats.

With each cycle, Non REM sleep becomes progressively lighter, and REM sleep becomes progressively longer, lasting from a few minutes early in sleep to perhaps an hour at the end of the sleep episode.

People with Sleep apnea usually do not remember waking up during the night. Indications of the problem may be such vague symptoms as excessive daytime sleepiness; morning headache; irritability; impaired mental or emotional functioning; snoring (bed partners may report very loud and interrupted snoring); heartburn (acid back-up that causes heartburn, in fact, may be responsible for some cases of Sleep apnea.)

Any abnormality in the throat, mouth or nose that causes some obstruction in the upper airways and reduces air pressure can produce Sleep apnea syndrome. Among the most likely structural causes of many cases of Sleep apnea are abnormalities in the soft palate and surrounding throat walls that make them collapse more easily during breathing.

Chronic snoring itself may actually be a cause of some cases of Sleep apnea. Over time the vibrations and the increased pressure against the upper airways as snoring people inhale may cause the soft palate to lengthen. This stretched palate is more prone to collapse and obstruction. It should be stressed that snoring is very common. It does not always cause apnea nor is it always a sign of the respiratory disorder. Snoring is also associated with daytime sleepiness regardless of whether apneas are present but snoring alone does not appear to pose any major health risks.)

Obesity is strongly associated with sleep apnea and there is some evidence it may be a cause of it. Imaging scans have shown fatty cells infiltrating the throat tissue, which suggest that they could narrow the airways. One study showed the more obese a person with sleep apnea was, the higher the pressure on the airway and therefore the greater the obstruction of the airway.

GERD (the cause of heartburn) may be a cause of Sleep apnea. With this disorder, stomach acid backs up into the esophagus. This event can produce spasms of the vocal cords (larynx), thereby blocking the flow of air to the lungs.

Some researchers estimate that 18 to 25 million people have sleep apnea, but less than a million are aware of it. More men than women appear to have sleep apnea. Sleep apnea may be under-diagnosed in women. In general, older women have the same incidence as men their own age. A range of studies has reported Apnea or hypopnea in between 9% and 24% of men and in 4% to 15% of women.

Sleep apnea affects people of all ages. Although it is most common in older adults, it has been reported in between 1.6% to 3.4% of children. Some experts believe that sleep disorder breathing may occur in as many as 11% of children. Interestingly, one study suggested that although prevalence of Sleep apnea increases with age, its health consequences decline. In the study, Apnea posed more of a threat to a person's health before age 45 than afterward.

Often, body position greatly affects the number and severity of episodes of Obstructive Sleep Apnea, with at least twice as many Apneas occurring when a person lies face upward than when the person lies on his or her side. This may be due to the effects of gravity, which cause the throat to narrow when a person lies on his or her back. Smokers are at higher risk for Apnea, with heavy smokers (more than 2 packs a day) having a risk 40 times greater than nonsmokers. Alcohol use has been associated with Apnea, although studies are mixed. A major 1999 survey reported that 53% of people who use alcohol experience symptoms of sleep apnea. One study found no relationship.

As many as 200,000 automobile accidents in the US and 1,500 deaths from such accidents are caused by sleepiness. Studies continue to report that drowsy driving is as risky as drunk driving.

Estimates on fatigue as a cause of automobile crashes range from 1% to 56%, depending on the study. A large 1997 survey indicated that accidents involving motor vehicles or machine tools occurred twice as often in persons with moderate or severe daytime sleepiness, compared with those without daytime sleepiness.

In a major 1995 poll, 33% of those surveyed said they had fallen asleep while driving and 10% of these people had had accidents because of this.

One study found that older people with Sleep apnea and daytime sleepiness have lower scores on tests for cognitive functions.

One expert suggested that treating Sleep apnea in older patients may correct some cases of dementia that are caused by sleep disturbances. Elderly people with Sleep apnea may also be more prone to depression.

For some people, sleep disorders, including Apnea, may be the underlying causes of some chronic headaches. In some patients with both chronic headaches and Apnea, treating the sleep disorder has been known to cure the headache, even a cluster headache in one case.

The effects of Sleep apnea on major health conditions are currently under debate. Among the problems that have been associated with this sleep disorder are:

i) High blood pressure;

ii) Stroke;
iii) Heart attack;
iv) Heart failure;
v) Pulmonary Hypertension;
vi) Diabetes;
vii) Kidney failure.

Researchers are intensively investigating why a problem in the upper airways is associated with these serious health events. Obesity, smoking and alcohol abuse, known risk factors for hypertension and heart disease, are also associated with Sleep apnea. These factors however, do not explain all cases of higher heart risk in people with Sleep apnea. For example, among overweight people, those who have Sleep apneas have a greater heart risk than those without them. When breathing stops during Apneas, carbon dioxide levels in the blood increase and oxygen levels drop. This effect may trigger a cascade of physical and chemical events that can then increase risk for these conditions.

Researchers have reported high levels of certain immune factors called tumor necrosis factor-alpha (TNF-alpha) and interleukin 6 (IL-6) in people with Sleep apnea, particularly those who are obese. High levels of TNF-alpha and IL-6 produce a damaging inflammatory response, which can harm cells in the body, including those in the arteries. Elevated TNF-alpha was associated in one study with fatigue, shortness of breath, and a weak heart-pumping action.

At this time, however, evidence of a clear causal relationship with any of these health problems is still weak. Some studies have found no significant independent risk for heart disease from Obstructive Sleep Apnea. The following are some discussions on the possible effects of apnea on specific health problems.

A number of studies have found a strong association between Sleep apnea and high blood pressure (hypertension). For example, a 2000 study followed patients for four years and reported that the greater the number of nightly Apnea episodes they had in year one the more likely they were to develop hypertension by the fourth year. A weak but still higher than normal association with high blood pressure has even been observed in those who snore or have mild Sleep apnea.

The relationship between Sleep apnea and hypertension has been thought to be largely due to obesity, a risk factor common to both conditions. Recent and major studies, however, are suggesting a higher rate of hypertension in people with Sleep apnea regardless of weight.

The following is one way that Apnea may directly affect blood pressure, regardless of other risk factors:

Blood pressure fluctuates widely and suddenly in response to episodes of Apnea and hypopnea. Such fluctuations are possibly due to a sudden surge in the sympathetic nervous system, which has also been associated with Sleep apnea. The sympathetic nervous system controls involuntary muscles, importantly those in the blood vessels and heart.

Over time such fluctuations could possibly lead to permanent hypertension.

Sleep apnea appears to increase the chance for a stroke independent of its association with high blood pressure, a known risk factor for stroke. Sleep apnea is also thought to be related to small strokes called transient ischemic attacks (TIAs). How Sleep apnea increases these risks is under investigation. Some theories include: that blood becomes more viscous (stickier) in the morning in people with Obstructive Sleep Apnea compared to people without the sleep disorder. Such "sticky" blood is more apt to form clots that can lead to stroke. Stroke victims with Sleep apnea tended to have higher levels of the blood protein fibrinogen than stroke victims without Sleep apnea. Fibrinogen is a factor in blood that causes it to clot. Higher levels of fibrinogen have been linked to both stroke and heart attack risk.

A 1998 study reported that the carotid artery (the major artery to the brain) is in far greater danger of becoming *sclerotic* (hardening and narrowing) in people with Obstructive Sleep Apnea than in the average person. People with both diabetes and Sleep apnea are at particularly high risk for this effect.

One small 1998 study reported a drop in blood flow in the brain during episodes of obstructive hypopnea (slow and shallow breathing associated with snoring). This may also contribute to the risk of stroke. Such declines in blood flow did not appear to occur with obstructive or central *Apnea*, however.

Researchers observed that the higher the number of Apneas and hypopneas a patient had, the higher his risk for heart attack. Many of the factors associated with stroke and Sleep apnea (a risk for blood clots and narrowing of the arteries) may also increase the risk for heart attacks. Evidence suggests, however, that the effect of Apneas on coronary artery disease and heart attack is not as significant as it is on heart failure and stroke.

The evidence of an association between heart failure and Sleep apnea is suggested by:

High blood pressure, which is associated with Sleep apnea, is a major cause of later heart failure; Apneas in patients with left ventricular hypertrophy. This is an overgrowth of the heart's left ventricle that impairs the heart's pumping action over time and is a major factor in many cases of heart failure (more research is needed to verify these results); Central Sleep Apnea is particularly linked with heart failure. In any case, Obstructive Sleep Apnea can affect breathing functions in a way that may be particularly harmful for patients with existing congestive heart failure. A 1999 study, in fact, indicated that Sleep apnea is associated with poorer survival in patients with heart failure.

Researchers have also observed an association between diabetes and Sleep apnea. Obesity may be the common factor, but there is also some evidence that Sleep apnea is associated with abnormalities in insulin regulation independent of other conditions.

Obstructive Sleep Apnea can play a role in the development of pulmonary hypertension, a serious but uncommon condition in which pressure rises in the blood vessels in the lungs.

Other Physical Effects of Sleep apnea:

Irregular menstrual periods accompany Apnea in about 40% of pre-menopausal women. It is not clear how they are related, but one study reported that treating Apnea helped normalize periods.

Patients with Sleep apnea also appear to be at higher risk for glaucoma, a serious eye condition related to nerve damage in the optic nerve. One theory for this association is that the drop in blood oxygen that occurs during Apneas may either damage the nerve directly or increase pressure in the eye, a cause of glaucoma.

Studies report an association between severe Apnea and psychological problems. In one study, 32% of patients had symptoms of depression. Certainly, daytime sleepiness interferes with quality of life. It is also possible that severe emotional problems might worsen the Apnea. One study investigated the effects of the antidepressant paroxetine (Paxil) on patients with Obstructive Sleep Apnea. The agent improved breathing during late sleep stages but had little effect on other aspects of Obstructive Sleep Apnea.

Because Sleep apnea so often includes noisy snoring, the condition can also adversely affect the sleep quality of a patient's bed-partner. Spouses or partners may also suffer from sleeplessness and fatigue. In some cases, the snoring can even disrupt relationships. Diagnosis and treatment of Sleep apnea in the patient can, of course, help eliminate these problems.

People who habitually snore and have observable breathing irregularities, even if they are *not* sleepy during the day, in some cases, may need to consult a sleep specialist. At most, sleep disorders centers' patients undergo an in-depth analysis, usually supervised by a multi-disciplinary team of consultants who can provide both physical and psychiatric evaluations. In the U.S., one night at a sleep clinic costs about $1,200 to $1,600 and is not always covered by insurance. In Canada, we are fortunate enough to have such an evaluation covered by our provincial medical insurance.

As a first step in dealing with Sleep apnea, the patient should simply try rolling over onto the side. Patients who sleep on their backs and have 50 to 80 Apneas (breathless events) per hour can sometimes reduce them to nearly zero when they shift to one side or the other. The more overweight a person is, the less effective changing positions is, but it still helps.

Some suggestions that might help a person maintain a low-risk sleeping position are as follows:

- Sew a small pocket to the back of the pajamas and place a tennis or other small ball into it.
- More expensive products, including a gravity-triggered alarm, are available.
- A special pillow that helps to stretch the neck may reduce snoring and improve sleep for people with mild Sleep apnea.

One study suggested that sleeping in an upright position could improve oxygen levels in overweight people with Sleep apnea.

Over-the-counter nasal strips may significantly improve early-stage sleep in people with sleep disorders associated with nasal obstruction. They are not intended as treatments for sleep apnea, however.

All overweight patients with Obstructive Sleep Apnea should attempt a weight-reducing program. Weight loss certainly reduces snoring in many people, sometimes stopping it completely. Although few well-conducted studies have been performed to determine the effects of weight loss on Apnea itself, one 2000 study suggested that people who lost 10% of body weight experienced an average 26% reduction in risk for developing Sleep apnea. Gaining 10% of their body weight, on the other hand, increased the odds of Sleep apnea. In any case, losing weight is certainly important for healthy blood pressure and for reducing the risk for diabetes.

The following tips are useful for patients who use or abuse alcohol, cigarettes, sleeping pills, or any combination:

- Smokers should quit.
- Alcohol should be avoided within four hours of sleep.
- In general, drugs have not been very beneficial except for specific situations.

Sedatives and anti-anxiety drugs can actually worsen the breathing disturbances and arousal conditions that occur with Sleep apnea. These substances cause the soft tissues in the throat to sag and diminish the body's ability to inhale. Apnea sufferers should stay away from sleeping pills and tranquilizers completely.

At this time, the most effective treatments for Sleep apnea are devices that deliver slightly pressurized air to keep the throat open during the night. There are a number of variations available. The treatment depends on the specific problems causing obstruction and their location. In order to determine the appropriate amount of air pressure, the patient usually needs to be monitored in a sleep laboratory. Although this may require only one night, patients may need to be retested if they do not experience improved daytime alertness.

Currently, the best treatment for severe obstructive and mixed Sleep apnea is a system known as nasal continuous positive airflow pressure (CPAP). It is safe and effective in Sleep apnea patients of all ages, including children and works in the following way: The device itself is a machine weighing about five pounds that fits on a bedside table; a mask containing a tube connects to the device and fits over just the nose; the machine supplies a steady stream of air through a tube and applies sufficient air pressure to prevent the tissues from collapsing during sleep. All patients should be warned that the first few nights of CPAP therapy are unnerving. The device, particularly the mask, often produces anxiety, primarily because of the mask. Starting out with low pressure to get used to the mask may help. Patients may actually experience less sleep or sleep of a different quality in the beginning.

Nearly all patients complain about at least one side effect and nearly half of complaints are related to the mask. Many can be alleviated with a well-chosen mask that is comfortable and reduces leakage as much as possible. Chinstraps, nasal saline sprays or humidifiers may prevent these side effects. Heated humidification devices are also now available for CPAP users. Excessive application of pressure makes exhalation difficult.

A feeling of claustrophobia is a major factor in noncompliance, which may be alleviated with a lightweight and transparent mask or with masks known as nasal pillows, which are used only around the nostrils. Up to 30% of patients experience irritation and sores over the bridge of the nose. Getting a properly fitted and cushioned mask can help reduce this effect; eye irritation can occur; patients may also experience chest muscle discomfort for a while, which is caused by an increase in lung volume.

There have been reports of severe side effects, including heart arrhythmias, severe nose bleeding, and air pockets in the skull. These complications are very rare, however, and occur in only a few patients out of thousands.

Even after using CPAP for an average of only four hours a night, many patients report the following effects:

- Greater alertness;
- Less daytime sleepiness;
- Better concentration;
- Better mood.

In fact, if patients do not experience less sleepiness after a period of time and are still complying with the regimen, then the airflow pressure may not be high enough. Patients may require retesting. It should be noted that patients generally report feeling more alert after CPAP treatments, although laboratory tests may not show significant differences in number of Apneas or wake-up periods.

A 1999 study reported that work performance improved after six months of use.

A 1997 study indicated that CPAP therapy may even reduce the risks of motor vehicle and domestic and work-related accidents associated with sleepiness.

There is some evidence that this therapy may even help reduce abdominal fat, even if patients fail to lose weight. To date, there are no well-designed studies to indicate if any of these devices improve survival in patients with heart problems or other disorders associated with Sleep apnea. Improvement in serious conditions relating to the heart, such as hypertension and heart failure, has been observed in some studies, although the effect at least on high blood pressure has sometimes been small.

Bi-level Positive Airway Pressure systems (BiPAP) appear to be particularly helpful for patients with coexisting lung disease and those with excessive levels of carbon dioxide. These devices have a sensing feature that helps determine and vary the appropriate pressure depending on whether a person is breathing in or out. Greater pressure is needed on inhalation and less on exhalation. These machines are more expensive than the CPAP and may not be covered by insurance.

Even more sophisticated systems are available called auto-CPAP devices, which use greater technological capacity to customize air pressure. They usually employ one of three methods:

Overall pressure is kept low until a specific problem is detected. At that time the pressure is automatically increased rapidly.

Pressure is low when there are no problems but is raised gradually when they are detected.

Pressure is gradually raised and lowered in response to problems or their absence. In addition, the device can change depending on problems within single breaths.

Brands include AutoAdjust, Virtuoso, and AutoSet. These devices are more expensive than those that provide continuous airflow. And, in general, the pressure exerted using these devices is lower than with standard CPAP and there is little difference in effectiveness. These devices may improve compliance, however, in patients who find the steady flow of air from standard devices annoying or who require varying levels of pressure due to other conditions, such as seasonal allergies. They are also proving to be very useful as home diagnostic tools for Sleep apnea.

Several different dental appliances or treatments are available and are proving to be very valuable treatments for mild to moderate Obstructive Sleep Apnea. Dentists and orthodontists are slowly becoming more aware of Obstructive Sleep Apnea, and may become more involved with its diagnosis and treatment.

One common device is a splint that holds the tongue in a specific position to keep the airway as open as possible.

- Some dental devices are similar in appearance to sports mouth guards. The mandibular advancement device (MAD) forces the lower jaw forward, which keeps the airway open. Studies generally indicate satisfaction with the dental devices, although it is not known if they have any significant health benefits. Studies have indicated that MAD has the following benefits:
- It reduces Apneas significantly for those with mild to moderate Apnea, particularly if patients sleep on their backs.
- It may improve airflow, although less well, in those with severe Apnea.
- In one study 88% of patients rate their mandibular devices as "effective."
- It appears to improve sleep.

There are some disadvantages to this treatment:
- Dental devices are not as effective as CPAP therapy, but patients may be more satisfied with them.

- MAD generally has only minor and infrequent adverse effects, although a few patients experience pain in the jaw.
- In one study, patients who used dental devices reported less contentment after one year of use than those who had had *uvulopalatopharyngoplasty*, the standard Apnea surgery.
- In a small percentage of patients, the treatment may worsen Apnea. Patients should be monitored with *polysomnography* before and after therapy.

An orthodontic treatment called rapid maxillary expansion may be beneficial for patients with Sleep apnea and a narrow upper jaw. This non-surgical procedure takes about three weeks and helps to reduce nasal pressure and improve breathing. Surgery is sometimes recommended, usually by throat specialists. A patient should be sure to seek a second opinion from a specialist in sleep disorders. Few randomized clinical trials, the gold standard of medical research, have been conducted to verify the long-term efficacy of Sleep apnea surgery.

Surgery known as uvulopalatopharyngoplasty (UPPP) involves removing soft tissue on the back of the throat and palate. It may use cauterization or laser surgery. If tonsils are present, they are removed. The object of UPPP is threefold:

1. To increase the width of the airway at the throat's opening.
2. To block some of the muscle action in order to improve the ability to open.
3. To "square off" the soft palate to improve its movement and closure.

Uvulopalatopharyngoplasty is recommended only for select patients with severe Obstructive Sleep Apnea.

Success rates for Sleep apnea procedures are rarely higher than 65% and often are lower, averaging about 50% over the long-term.

The procedure also has a number of potentially serious complications. In fact, in one study, 42% of patients had complaints about the procedure. Some complications include the following:

- Infection. (In one study this complication was so common that 40% of patients needed another operation because of it.) Preventive antibiotics administered an hour before surgery can help reduce this risk.
- Mucus in the throat.
- Changes in voice frequency.
- Swallowing problems.
- Impaired sense of smell.
- Failure and recurrence of Apnea. In such cases, continuous positive airway pressure (CPAP) is often less effective afterward, although one study found that oral appliances may still help.

In one review of studies, 20% of patients who had UPPP required tracheostomy afterward. Most complications can be avoided with proper techniques and experienced surgeons. The use of lasers with UPPP is being investigated.

Tracheostomy used to be the only treatment for Sleep apnea. It is quite straightforward: The surgeon makes an opening through the neck into the windpipe and inserts a tube. It is almost 100% successful, but it requires a quarter-size opening in the throat. This produces a number of medical and psychological problems associated with recovery. Today, this is performed rarely, usually only if Sleep apnea is life-threatening. A new procedure that uses only a tiny opening may prove to be a good alternative.

A technique called radiofrequency ablation is of interest. It uses radio waves emitted from an electrode to treat patients who snore. The radio waves destroy a small amount of tissue at the base of the tongue. The therapy takes about twenty minutes and typically requires 10 treatments within five or six sessions. A newer form requires fewer treatment sessions because it provides more concentrated radio waves, and it appears to be effective. The procedure causes some discomfort, which can be controlled with simple pain relievers. It is far less invasive than standard surgery, and studies are reporting significant improvement in reduced snoring and less daytime sleepiness. It may be helpful for mild Obstructive Sleep Apnea.

Other procedures may be appropriate to correct facial abnormalities or throat obstructions that cause Sleep apnea. They may be used alone or combined with each other or with UPPP. Some patients with Obstructive Sleep Apnea have nasal obstructions (such as a deviated septum) that contribute to snoring and other symptoms. Surgery for such obstruction may be helpful in reducing symptoms and improving oxygen levels, although it does not always cure the condition.

CHAPTER 5: FISH OIL AND THE BRAIN

When I was first admitted to the hospital, I was diagnosed with a hemorrhagic bleed. Some ten days later, I had a second bleed and required emergency surgery to clear the blood clot in my brain and to drain the excess fluid that was accumulating and putting pressure on my brain.

As a child, I had been diagnosed as a hemophiliac although the condition was only apparent in the event of surgery or trauma above my neck. This included tooth extractions, injury to my gums and, of course, my hemorrhagic bleed. In cases where I had been injured or cut in any other place such as on my hand, foot or leg, my wounds always healed quickly and normally.

When Hélène and I recently went to the Health Food store to purchase a bottle of fish oil capsules, the clerk told us that she had read that fish oil increases the flow of blood and should therefore not be taken by hemophiliacs! She suggested we double-check this with either a pharmacist or our family physician. Hélène went to the pharmacy that very day and, upon checking in her medical books, the pharmacist confirmed that there is "a chance" that fish oil can increase the flow of blood. She suggested we go to our family physician to confirm one way or the other, which we did the other day. He advised us that using this product was of no concern in my particular situation. Better to be safe than sorry, I always say!

High-dose fish oil increases serotonin production which is the key for increasing the brain's threshold for stress. This is the same mechanism that some popular pharmaceutical drugs use to improve the mood of individuals. Fish oil is composed of long chained Omega-3 fatty acids. If these are removed from our diets, our leering ability is severely diminished. DHA is the key component in fish oil that our brains feed on. Supplementing our diets with a pharmaceutical grade fish oil supplement will ensure that our brains have the adequate resources of DHA (Docosahexaenoic Acid) to function at peak levels. An association between the brain content of DHA and mental capacity and health has recently been found. Studies have shown that when an individual consumes a highly stable form of fish oil, such as pharmaceutical grade fish oil or ultra refined omegarx fish oil, there is an increase in the concentration of DHA in the brain.

For example, children with lower levels of Omega-3 fatty acids have a lower mental capacity overall. The decrease is especially evident in studies involving mathematical problems, and these same children have difficulty sleeping and waking in the mornings. Studies have shown that when these children are given a pharmaceutical grade or ultra refined fish oil supplement, which is rich in DHA (one of the two essential fat components of fish oil), an increase in intellectual functions and capacity can be apparent in as little as two hours after consumption.

Certain mental problems are also associated with a decrease of serotonin levels in the brain. This diminished concentration is directly associated with the plasma levels of Omega-3 fatty acids, in particular DHA. This, along with the account of many other factors, suggests that fish oil is very important for proper and perhaps even heightened brain function.

Note that if you are looking for fish oil to supplement your diet, the importance of using a product that is pharmaceutical grade cannot be emphasized enough. There are many companies which promote different kinds of essential fatty acid supplements but few of them actually offer truly pharmaceutical grade fish oil. Ultra-refined fish oil is also a new emerging standard that is even purer and free of toxins. You would need to look for a product that is independently tested by a third party. The manufacturing company should be happy to volunteer their product to ensure product purity and safety. Also, you should look for a company that offers an unconditional guarantee because you, as a customer, are entitled to be satisfied under any circumstances. The most important variable associated with the supplementation of fish oil is to be free of toxins. Be sure to look for ultra-refined fish oil, pharmaceutical grade fish oil and third party independent lab testing.

Fish oil and fish oil supplements are considered by many to be the single most important missing component in diets today. It is an absolute necessity to arm ourselves with the best possible information on fish oil. Docosahexaenoic acid (DHA), an Omega-3 fatty acid, belongs to the class of nutrients called essential fatty acids.

DHA is one of the key essential fatty acids in fish oil. DHA's ability to pass through the threshold and enter the brain sets it apart from EPA, another Omega-3 fish oil that has also proved to be beneficial to the body. More than 60% of the weight of the brain is fat, and most of the long-chain Omega-3 fatty acids in the body are concentrated in the brain. Virtually all of this long-chained Omega-3 fat is in the form of DHA. The brain demands such high levels of DHA because it is critical for certain cell membranes such as the synapse (responsible for information transfer), the retina (for reception of visual inputs), and the mitochondria (to synthesize ATP). The key membrane cells cannot perform at peak levels without adequate DHA in their membranes. New neural connections cannot be made let alone maintenance of old ones. Fish oil is the most potent form of essential fatty acid available today.

DHA has been shown to reduce levels of blood triglycerides. High triglycerides are linked with heart disease in most, but not all, research. DHA alone appears to be just as effective as fish oils, which contain both DHA and eicosapentaenoic acid (EPA) in beneficially lowering triglyceride levels in people at risk for heart disease. In part, this may be because some DHA is converted to EPA in the body. Unlike EPA, however, DHA may not reduce excessive blood clotting.

DHA appears to be essential for normal visual and neurological (nervous system) development in infants. However, DHA supplementation did not affect the development of visual acuity in formula-fed infants in a double-blind trial. Nevertheless, other double-blind research links DHA supplementation in premature infants to better brain functioning. The effects of DHA on the nervous system may well extend beyond infancy. Young adults given 1.5 to 1.8 grams DHA per day showed less evidence of aggression in response to mental stress, compared with people in the control group in a double-blind trial.

DHA supplementation in healthy young men has been shown to decrease the activity of immune cells, such as natural killer (NK) cells and the cells that regulate inflammation responses in the body. The anti-inflammatory effects of DHA may be useful in the management of autoimmune disorders; however, such benefits need to be balanced with the potential for increased risk of infections.

DHA deficiency plays an important role in a group of congenital diseases called peroxisomal disorders, which damage the protective covering (myelin) around nerves. Although rare, the worst of these disorders (i.e., Zellweger's syndrome) is life-threatening within the first year of life. Daily oral supplementation of 100-600 mg of DHA has been shown to increase blood levels of DHA, to protect myelin, and to improve the signs and symptoms of these potentially devastating disorders.

Cold-water fish, such as mackerel, salmon, herring, sardines, black cod, anchovies, and albacore tuna are rich sources of DHA and EPA. Similarly, cod liver oil contains large amounts of DHA and EPA. Certain microalgae contain DHA and are used as a vegetarian source of this nutrient in some supplements. Most fish oil supplements contain 12% DHA.

SECTION TEN – LET ME SAY THIS ABOUT THAT

CHAPTER 1: CUSTOMER SERVICE EXCELLENCE

Whether they are in business or in ordinary, everyday life, people should treat and regard others in the same manner that they themselves would like to be treated. Often enough, not only do you not get the appropriate service and courtesy from stores or shops with which you are trying to do business, but their staff can actually be downright rude to you. At times, they make it very clear through their body language that they don't appreciate or want your business. This is usually an easy situation to remedy! At times like this we, as consumers, just need to band together and simply walk away and, most importantly, leave our money in our pockets. The message should usually be very clear and the problem quickly rectified.

All of us have opportunities to experience customer service, usually a few times each week. We are exposed to it when we go to the bank or the convenience store. We get to test it in the drug store, grocery store and when we get on the bus. We also get to decide whether we got an acceptable greeting at the door of a car dealership when planning to spend thousands of dollars. They don't realize that, many times, serious potential customers have walked into a dealership, been turned off by the cold and blank stare they received, turned right around and walked out, only to drive out and go across the street and commit their $30k or $40k to a more anxious and zealous salesman at a more attuned dealership! Gosh, I have done this a few times myself, walking right back out, very frustrated and feeling like my money was not important or welcome. Hence the 0 to 2 rating in Peter Frost's '0 to 10 customer service rating' system.

Most of the time, you simply end up needing to make a quick, easy decision! You must decide whether to do business with them or go back to them again; you must also decide where to spend your hard-earned money. It's not just you either; it's also the dozens of people you're likely to refer to that particular business or the fairly large group of friends and acquaintances you'll end up talking to about how poorly you were treated. If you walk away with a bad taste in your mouth, you're bound to suggest to your friends that they should avoid doing business with that particular retailer again.

The commodity to which you will be entitled is that of either good or poor customer service.

When you have experienced something as catastrophic as a stroke, you learn to depend on a great many wonderful people. In my case, one such person is our dentist, Mark. He is an amazing man. He does the most incredible work on your teeth, just like a wizard. In fact, all the staff at Avalon Dental Care in Whitby is just so terrific that they could write an instruction manual on how to provide the most impressive and comprehensive customer service. You will want this book and you certainly want to sit in their chairs.

Here are my suggested key factors of customer service excellence:

1. Going the extra mile

Is the sales agent proving to you that they want your business and are they prepared to bend over backwards to earn your money and make you happy with your purchase?

2. No cost customer service

What can they do for you to make you happy with your purchase? Did they indicate that they were pleased to have had the opportunity to work with you?

3. Do they want the business?

Do they realize you could've gone elsewhere?

4. Brain damage and customer service

Do they realize the true implications of a handicap? I have been severely handicapped and will no longer tolerate being treated as a second class citizen. I am now also prepared to raise shit at a moment's notice if I have to, and I am not alone! I have received much support and agreement regarding many of the injustices against the disabled community almost every day and I am determined to ensure that this area is improved, thus making the world a better place. What everyone must realize is that any day, unfortunately, you could end up in a situation similar to mine and be facing a whole new nightmarish world with an endless series of challenges and injustices. Not to mention our beloved seniors and our increasingly aging population. There, but for the grace of God… as they say!

5. Peter's 1-10 scale rating system

This system works easily. A quick 1-10 rating helps you come to conclusions quickly and you can tell people you know which of the businesses you deal with deserve a 10 and which ones should get a 2. You can struggle with numbers between 2 and 9 to rate precisely how you feel about what your experience has just been with a particular business or you can give a 10 to indicate that you were impressed and will do business with them again or you can give them a 1 and not ever bother with them again. Of course, you can and will debate these scores with your friends and neighbours.

These factors, if followed diligently, will ensure the ultimate level of customer satisfaction resulting in a happier clientele, less frustration, fewer strokes, guaranteed repeat business and referrals and a happier world overall. The message must be delivered LOUD AND CLEAR!!

One of the most prominent, technology-driven vehicles of customer service today is that of a Contact Centre or Call Centre. Another such facility is called a Telemarketing Centre. In such instances, telephone–equipped, well-trained agents or associates interface with the public and potential or actual customers to either sell or support products in either a proactive or a responsive mode. Telemarketing has been given a bad rap over the past 10 or 20 years because the general public has been groomed to consider such calls intrusive, annoying, unsolicited and generally just unwanted.

Call Centres are designed to respond to incoming calls and are usually better understood and received by the public. Such calls are typically initiated by the customer, usually to place an order or request service, at a time that is satisfactory to them and such calls are therefore not unexpected or intrusive. It still remains absolutely essential that the completed transaction is a successful and pleasant experience for the customer; otherwise there can be a considerable waste of time and resources and certainly some lost goodwill and opportunity.

Case in point, The Tree Cutter: Recently, I had the opportunity to make arrangements to have two large trees cut down, an old maple and a Dutch elm. The maple tree was probably about 30 years old and about 80' tall. Both trees were located in our backyard, looming precariously above our 32' x 16' oval-shaped above-ground swimming pool. The maple tree, in particular, swayed threateningly high above our home's roof, above our pool and over the neighbour's roof behind us. The tree also constantly shed considerable debris, twigs, maple keys, branches, leaves and such into our pool from early May to late fall, when we finally closed the pool for the winter. We had discussed a few times that we wanted to remove the two trees, but always put the project on hold, mostly due to the cost.

On this one particular day, we were driving through our neighbourhood on the way to our Tai Chi class and we passed a tree-cutter's truck. His wood grinder and equipment were parked on the side of the road in front of a home in our neighbourhood. The gentleman who owned the equipment was in the process of cutting two trees down for the homeowner, whose house we were passing. On the way back from our class, my wife suggested that we stop and ask this tree-cutter to stop by our place and give us a price to cut down two trees in our yard. My wife got out of the van and went over and spoke to the homeowner standing there, who then immediately called the tree-cutter over. Poor Steve (the tree-cutter) had apparently been shimmying up and down the trees all day, because people kept stopping to ask him about other possible jobs! He gave us his business card and promised to come by later that day to quote on our work. The fellow whose house he was working at praised and recommended him highly and said that he had priced the job with several other companies and had determined that this was the best price he could get and that he was comfortable having him do work for him and very pleased with the job so far.

As promised, Steve came by our home at about 5:00 pm or so, checked over the work that needed to be done, what encumbrances he would have to deal with, etc. and gave us a price. He turned out to be one of the most personable, friendly and reliable people we have ever had the pleasure of dealing with! This man not only just wanted to do the job; he wanted to assure us that we would absolutely have no regrets doing business with him. This was a man who knew his way in life and was going to do well regardless of his undertaking!

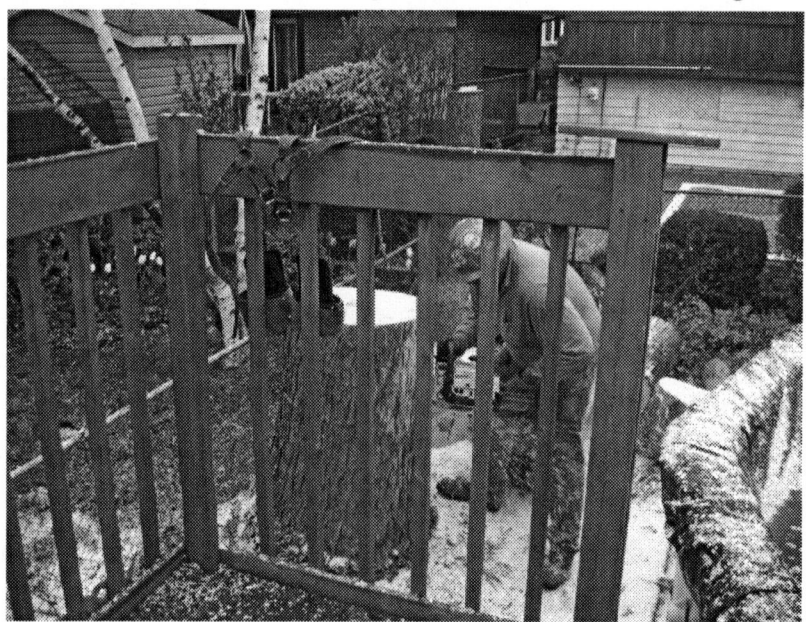

Steve, the tree cutter – Spring, 2005

That day, I tell you, was so spectacular. Steve capably climbed those 80' trees and skillfully took the assorted limbs and branches down and performed for the neighbourhood for the whole day. Occasionally, we would yell up and joke with him as the day progressed, all the time Steve and his crew being personable and having and taking the time to assure us that we had made the right decision to do business with him.

His final wrap up was the most incredible experience of customer service and satisfaction that I can ever recount in my thousands of opportunities for good customer service that I can recall. Steve still had to cut and pile the branches and sections of trunk that were now strewn around the property. The next morning, he came over and proceeded to sweep every last bit of twigs and sawdust he had created the day before, repeatedly saying how much he appreciated the business.

He never stopped until the work site was actually cleaner than before he had come over and begun the work. One of our neighbours, Mark and his son, Luke, 7, even came by to watch the spectacle and ended up helping stack some of the logs. Well, all the time, Steve never ceased telling us how much he appreciated having the business, and even then, never stopped picking up and cleaning up as he chatted and answered our questions and told us of some of his business adventures after the major work was done. His crew, Rob and Ryan were much the same. They were the absolute epitome of efficiency, courtesy and professionalism which was simply the only way Steve knew how to and wanted to work!

Steve is a '10' in my 1-10 customer service rating system and deserves much success in life and in his future endeavours. It was indeed an absolute pleasure! Good luck to you, Steve. You will enjoy much success with no sleepless nights. Why is it that some other people just don't get it?

Another wonderful story I have to share is one about people, humanity and simply just plain old fashioned good neighbours! Quite often, moving to a great neighbourhood is simply ordinary good luck, nothing more. For example, you could buy a new home or rent an apartment that took you months to find, only to discover the neighbour likes to play their stereo full-blast until 1:00 am every night, or likes to hold skinny dip parties in their pool or hot tub that your kid's bedroom window overlooks or always decides to cut their lawn on days after you have been working late and want/need to get some serious rest. Of course, there are situations when you just never have an issue and there are times when you will cut your neighbours' section of grass between your houses, or you will discover they have cut yours. Also, there is, of course, the communal tool inventory. Why would everyone on the block need to buy a 'whipper snipper' or a 'pressure washer'?

Almost three years ago, we purchased a new home in a charming neighbourhood and were in the process of painting the bedrooms before our furniture was delivered and moved in. Before we realized it, our front lawn had filled with a good number of our new neighbours, welcoming us to the neighbourhood. They greeted us with a computer printout of their first and last names, their kids' names and their addresses and phone numbers. We keep a copy of the list on our fridge and it has contributed to our comfort with the neighbourhood and has helped everyone know each other and stay in touch. This certainly lends itself to a friendlier and warmer neighbourhood!

Also, the neighbours on our street have become inclined to keep an eye on each other's homes when any of us is either away on vacation or just out for the evening. This has resulted in a safer and more secure neighbourhood and lifestyle, not to mention adding to the overall property value. Yes, we consider ourselves to be pretty lucky! In fact, these wonderful new neighbours proved themselves to us in a major way when I had my stroke. Even though we had only been in the house for less than six months (and during the winter at that, when people really don't socialize that often), many of them rallied around my wife and boys to do whatever they could to help. They did odd jobs around the property. *Thanks, Bill, for cleaning our eaves troughs without us ever even asking!* Dave helped Hélène open and close our pool just after my stroke, the first summer we were in the house. Dave often helps us with short notice emergency jobs, without any expectation on his part. *Thanks, Dave. You're awesome!* Others gave Hélène a shoulder to cry on when I was in hospital and things were so uncertain. Some occasionally invited her over for a drink or for dinner. *Thanks, Dave and Theresa! Your support was and is so appreciated. You are truly what wonderful, supportive neighbours are all about!* Still others were just there to listen and offer whatever assistance they could such as drive Tyler to his night classes; drive Hélène to the train station or pick her up at the end of her visit with me. *Thanks so much Maralynne and Karen!* All in all, we are surrounded by some of the best people we have ever encountered and they were virtual strangers to us when all this started.

Yet another very positive experience I had was when my wife and I recently went shopping for a freezer. We happened to be in a Home Depot outlet a few weeks ago and decided to stop by the Appliance Department to see what they had as our small fridge was now melting things in the freezer compartment and freezing things in the refrigerator. The salesman there, by the name of Eamon, could not have been more cordial and helpful. By the time we left the store, he had agreed to deliver the new freezer to us and take away our old fridge at no charge!

It took us a couple of weeks to actually order the freezer. When we finally did, over the phone, Eamon remembered us and was very accommodating. The freezer was delivered, as promised, four days later and the old fridge was hauled away. Then the incident happened: You see, our garage has a second garage door opening out to the backyard. The delivery company placed the new freezer at the back of the garage, near the door, as requested. Unfortunately however, none of us noticed that the ballast arm of the garage door would potentially hit and scrape the freezer when the door was opened!

About an hour or so after the delivery truck left, my wife and I were out in the garage admiring our new purchase and I asked her to open the back garage door so I could wheel myself through and into the back yard. As the BBQ was in front of the door, Hélène went in to the house and around to the back, moved the BBQ and attempted to open the garage door. It wouldn't open easily so, naturally, she assumed that something on the outside was blocking it. She moved a small table we had out there and tried again. Still, it wouldn't open! So she gave it a good heave... only to realize (too late) that the new freezer, inside, was blocking the door! So here we now are, with a wonderful brand new freezer, severely scratched and dented!

Well, never let it be said that I'm a slouch or a pushover! I immediately called Home Depot to report the incident and unfortunately found that Eamon was off that day. However, the fellow who answered the phone in the Appliance Department listened to my story and clearly wanted to contribute to this customer's complete satisfaction. He suggested that I would have to call the customer service department of the manufacturer (Maytag). He gave me the telephone number and I immediately gave them a call. Their position was that they unfortunately could not assume responsibility and we should talk to the local distributor, Home Depot. So... I called Home Depot back! Once again, I spoke to someone other than Eamon. The salesman, whose name was Mike, listened to my story and politely said that he would get back to me soon.

About two hours later, Mike called me back. He had contacted Maytag and had been told basically the same thing as I had been. Not taking no for an answer, he called Eamon AT HOME and told him the story. Eamon asked Mike to call me back and tell me that he (Eamon) would look after things when he came back in to work in a couple of days. He assured me that the freezer would be replaced with a new one and that they would simply use ours as a floor model (of the scratch and dent variety!). Now talk about true customer service! This store's practice and policy was to make sure that we, the customer, had a successful experience with their company. In my books, according to Peter's "customer service rating system", Eamon and Home Depot also deserve a "10"!

And to top this all off, the story of Home Depot's customer service doesn't just end there. A few weeks ago, Hélène and I found ourselves back there needing to make yet another 'special order purchase'. Well, it seems that their 'go the extra mile' customer service is not just a fluke 'shot in the dark' method of doing business. This time, we were in need of a 'special order' medicine cabinet. It was an obviously particularly busy Friday evening and our sales girl, Amber, was being bombarded with questions and requests from various other customers and staff. We had fortunately managed to secure her attention and she was extremely patient and was obviously not about to leave us in the lurch, answering our every question and making steady progress in placing our order. Before long, our order was placed and Amber had given us a satisfactory delivery date and we walked out of yet another pleasant experience with Home Depot.

Another 10 for Amber and Home Depot!

The list of these wonderful experiences goes on and on. Adrian and Nancy have become very good friends of ours in the past year or so. That relationship developed over an interesting sequence of circumstances. As I was just describing how we met Steve, the tree-cutter and how he did such an excellent job for us and how his customer service was 'second-to-none', well, one day, Hélène and I were reviewing our growing list of jobs around the house that needed doing. For the most part, the list consisted of jobs that required an able bodied person with two good arms and hands.

Anyway, the list was looking ugly! Homeownership can be and, in fact is a wonderful thing. Whether it's a new home or a 'handy-man special', there will always be little things that you require or need to do or get done in order to make it your special 'castle', to say nothing of the repairs that always come up when you own a house.

In this case, we had put together a sizeable "To Do" list of a growing number of jobs that we felt we needed and would like to get done around the house. In previous years, it was usually taken for granted that I would do these jobs. Why not? I had the knowledge, the experience and all the hand tools, power tools and more that a typical homeowner would have or need. In fact, over the years I had built a few cottages, some recreation rooms, various pieces of furniture and had also performed the electrical, plumbing and the associated carpentry, dry wall, finishing and any painting that was required to complete the projects. At one time, I even partnered in and managed a small construction business. I had saved a small fortune over the years working on the five or six homes that I had owned.

Well, circumstances were different now and my impatience to get things done sooner than later and to our meticulous specifications was driving us crazy. We had budgeted to have reserves aside to allow us to keep our wonderful home in good repair and to effect miscellaneous improvements. However, common sense and affordability always had to prevail and we would carefully pick and choose (prioritize) our projects. We also are pretty shrewd and fussy shoppers. We want nice things but know that nice things cost money so we are selective and strategic when it comes to selecting our items and projects and when we are going to get them and do them. Every other item seems to end up coming from Home Depot, although we find the occasional specific need at Canadian Tire or Home Hardware.

So, in deciding we needed to get these things done, we decided that, since we had had such a positive experience dealing with Steve, we would ask him if he knew anyone who did handy-work and other such small jobs. When we asked him, he said that a friend of his, who was also his neighbour, had been a chef at a local private school and a dinner theatre and had just become unemployed and was looking to do some handyman work. Steve highly recommended Adrian, which was a good enough referral for us!

So, the next day, Steve came over with Adrian and introduced us to him. We discussed a few jobs we needed doing and he gave us some reasonable proposals and we hired him. Well, not unlike Steve's style and capability, he finished some work for us quickly and efficiently and at attractive costs. His professional personality and the quality of work have encouraged us to continue working with him and for us to recommend him highly to anyone we learn of who needs similar services. Again, we have been so fortunate to have met yet another superb source of customer service excellence and, to top it off, Adrian and his wife have also become wonderful friends of ours. Of course, I am hoping and expecting that some readers of this literary endeavour may and should become referrals for these marvelous entrepreneurs.

As we already knew and were satisfied with the type of work that Steve could do, we knew that we couldn't go wrong getting work done by anyone referred to us by him. Thanks, Steve! Thanks, Adrian!

And the referral and recommendation process continues… Hélène and I were recently remarking how our front and back yards were growing out of control. I used to enjoy household gardening before becoming disabled and could keep up with the grass, plants and shrubs but it was becoming obvious that professional assistance and experienced consultation would be required to establish and maintain an attractive landscape. So, once more we sought some experienced assistance and called and hired a landscape professional who was referred to us by Adrian, who happens to be her neighbour; we immediately got good quotes from Beata, who is turning out to be of the same breed as her two neighbours, as we have determined by the quality and work ethic we are experiencing from her. Thanks Beata!

By the way, here are the contact numbers for these amazing, personable experts:

☏ Steve: Expert Tree Service: Tree Service and Stump Grinding
905-666-0063

☏ Adrian: Falkirk Construction Group: Fencing, Renovations, Carpentry, Landscape Design, Handyman Services and General Construction
905-925-6294

☏ Beata: Garden Design by Beata
905-665-6294

Hopefully these references and experiences can save you some time, frustration and money.

CHAPTER 2: MY CUSTOMER SERVICE EXPERIENCE

During my working life, from 1973 to 2003, I worked for:

- an Ottawa area cable company [18 years];
- a national communications company [5 years];
- a music and video mail order company [6 years];
- a local energy company [1 year].

In this day and age, management that is afraid to lose control has enabled business environments of limited loyalty or commitment because there is no job security. What comes first, commitment or loyalty, dedication or security? What precipitates the other, performance or security? Where does dedication and commitment fit into these equations?

In the years of my employment experience, I learned how to maintain solid Customer Service teams through the effective use of motivation and recognition, combined with the appropriate threat and use of discipline including potential termination of employment, if necessary. I realize that this last inference is rather ominous and scary and potentially demoralizing however, try to imagine yourself in the position of any employer who is facing possible bankruptcy or closure or even a serious loss of market share to the competition because their employees just won't or can't do their bit to serve their customers properly. Picture the position of a 35 year old father of three children, 1 to 8 years, with a dedicated young wife and mother. They should be looking forward to paying down the family mid-size car and the mortgage on their first house. The young junior executive is busting his ass trying his best to do a fabulous job and make his superiors happy that he is able to contribute to a harmoniously productive work environment of which he can be proud to be a part. Yet, he has to look over at the guy next to him, who takes excessive coffee and smoke breaks and generally just slacks off and demonstrates a poor work ethic, frequently calling in sick, demonstrating a bad attitude and an overall ugly work disposition. This simply is just not right! The exercise of 'termination of employment' involves the use of legal and fair techniques to assist the employee and employer to make proper decisions about an appropriate employment status for him or herself and the company. Usually, employees who are not productive and cooperative are unhappy anyways. The key to this strategy is that you don't want to keep people who will compromise your business and devalue existing hard working teams because they will drag your business down very quickly. It simply is not fair to those who mean well, work hard and are committed to a sincere work ethic each and every working day.

It is not fair to good performers and the people you are trying to train to be valuable and hopefully help the business to keep those employees who simply won't or can't do their part. It is usually clear and apparent to everyone when certain employees don't do their share and the conclusion becomes obvious. This inferior conduct will spread like a disease. Also, it will be difficult to detect the actual source of the problem and it will be very costly to correct (termination, rehiring, retraining costs, etc.).

You cannot trust individuals who have a low or questionable sense of values. Poor performers will also not trust their bosses or perform honestly, because they know that their superiors can probably see right through them and may even have their number already. So they will probably try to take advantage at every opportunity, creating an atmosphere of dishonesty, mistrust and low morale.

The goal in every business has to be to work hard together as a team to win and keep customers. Companies and employees who have figured this out will and do deserve to succeed!

I learned this technique of *termination* from a former 'legal' associate with whom I worked on a series of interesting projects in the earlier part of my career. If an employee was obviously not happy with his/her employment and was not prepared to commit to his/her working association, he/she was better off severing his or her employment relationship altogether (or having it severed for him/her).

CHAPTER 3:   SLOW DOWN

Since I got sick and have had brain surgery and am now experiencing severe short-term memory impairment, I find that technological progress and development from a typical consumer's perspective is just racing past us at an incredible rate. In fact, despite my condition, I still have the awareness and interest in technology and marketing that allows me to be fascinated by the latest gadgets and digital accessories. Since regaining consciousness and proceeding with a rehab program for my stroke including physiotherapy and using an electro-stimulation bio-feedback device to help me with the paralysis of my arm, fingers and leg, I have learned about iPods, digital cameras, GPS units, MP3s, DVDs, etc. I even purchased a Palm Pilot to assist me with my memory deficit as I try to recall details of subject matter for my book and miscellaneous details of daily occurrences and conversations. Understanding that these toys have been available since as long ago as 1999 or so, I am only now actually becoming aware of them and familiar with their operation. It is all much like a dream. How quickly and how recently did all this technology evolve? How did it all seem to pass me by? Was I out with this sickness that long? It sure seems like a dream.

Another recent frustration has been with my current PC and Windows XP, replacing the earlier Microsoft operating systems. About a year and a half before having my stroke, we had purchased an upgraded, high memory, large capacity hard drive and high speed Celeron processor PC. We were of the impression that, replacing our 486, it would probably be all that we would need for a very long time. After my discharge from hospital and return home, I eventually started expressing an interest in getting back on the computer. Unbeknownst to me, while I was hospitalized Hélène had a series of problems with our PC and it had been recommended to her to upgrade to Windows XP. So, not only did I need to relearn the operation of the PC, I was also faced with learning a whole new operating system! Augh!!! My poor damaged brain!

I must say though that I persevered and, after relearning the basics as well as how to use MS Word, MS Excel, Yahoo Mail, MS Outlook Express and various other software packages that had been installed, I slowly and gradually found that I was able to be proficient at a keyboard once more, albeit without my left hand. During one of our Health Recovery Weeks last year, one of the other participants told me about an available keyboard feature that would change my life forever.

"Sticky Keys" is designed for people who have difficulty holding down two or more keys simultaneously. When a shortcut requires a combination of keys, such as CTRL+C, "Sticky Keys" will allow you to press the modifier key (CTRL, ALT, or SHIFT) and it will remain active until another key is pressed. This amazing tool allows a one-handed typist to be able to more readily and speedily negotiate the keyboard whenever they need to insert an Upper Case letter or perform any Control or Alt function.

To activate "Sticky Keys," open "Accessibility Options" in the "Control Panel" of your Windows PC; on the "Keyboard" tab, under "Sticky Keys," select the "Use Sticky Keys" checkbox.

As you can see, I have been able to produce this book! Recently, Hélène bought me a laptop for Father's Day, my next few birthdays, the next few Christmases, etc. as a much needed tool to assist me with writing this and the next few such projects.

In fact, interestingly enough, about three years after my stroke and about one year after starting to type on a keyboard again and work on my book, I am starting to experience considerable pain in my "good" right hand. It appears that I am over-using my right hand and even my physiotherapists have pointed out astutely that I obviously have to use my right knee for everything, because of my left-side paralysis and that I should give my right side "a break" once in a while too. I want to thank the therapists at the Whitby Day Hospital for encouraging me to give my right side a much needed vacation! It worked! I am noticing that the pain is far less severe than it was a few weeks ago.

SECTION ELEVEN – FROM ME TO YOU

CHAPTER 1: PERSEVERANCE IS THE BEST MEDICINE

It is an interesting challenge to try to write a book with the brain damage I have had, because it is almost impossible to remember where one thought ends and another one begins. There is no question I am lucky to be alive, having endured such devastation to my mental and physical being.

I have become compelled to want to express this experience in type for others because it has been an unfortunate and inescapable nightmare that often feels as though there will be no salvation. As I type away with my one good hand, I feel dizzy and like I am going to fall forward. My physio and occupational therapists constantly remind me to sit up straight to try and maintain my posture. So every once in a while, I do sit up straight to help overcome a sensation of falling and it helps me feel a little more in control of my destiny. I also always enjoy a good stretch and to get away from my tendency to slouch.

With the brain damage that I have, it is difficult for me to try to assemble my thoughts. After all, I had surgery on my brain at the back of my head in the area of my cerebellum that has left me with extreme dizziness and difficulty concentrating.

It is so important to me that I recognize and warmly thank my wonderful, loving wife whom I am so lucky to constantly have by my side as she always cares for me. She has helped me with the editing of this book that I could never have completed alone with the partial brain function with which

I am left. However, using my personal computer, I am able to put my thoughts down in front of me and I am better able to recall, organize and assemble them in a logical sequence. As I attempt to write this book, which has been so therapeutic and challenging for me, it just feels so great to be able to put these complex thoughts and ideas together! However, as I sit at my keyboard, I am wrestling with themes and trying to capture and remember them as I get through assembling a few key thoughts.

Fortunately, my wife and I both have a pretty strong grasp of grammar, punctuation and spelling. Hélène has helped me edit and proofread this manuscript and I have been able to make progress through most of the thoughts with little difficulty and within a reasonable amount of time.

It is now early in the summer of 2006 and I am still not yet walking normally. However, I have come a long way, a long way from where I was when I first had my stroke during the winter of 2003. When I had my stroke on February 17, 2003, I was rendered comatose, fell unconscious on the bathroom floor, fortunately was immediately discovered by my wife, tended to and rushed to the hospital. When I awoke, I began my *Long, Challenging Journey*.

I soon found out that this tragic medical emergency had left me paralyzed on the left side, with brain surgery that resulted in serious impairment to my short-term memory and an incessant, numbing pain that took over my entire left side. I could not walk, nor could I use or even move my left hand. I was not going to be able to play anymore gigs with my band-mates. For the next three years to this time in 2006, I was to wake up daily with a painful extreme stiffness in my left leg and arm. I took physiotherapy three times a week for the first couple of years and reduced that to twice a week as recently as April of this year.

Today I am walking with a side walker and am determined to walk normally again. My physiotherapy, combined with stimulating and calming Taoist Tai Chi, has strengthened my limbs and muscles to the point that I am able to stand, bear weight on my left leg and foot, as well as on my left arm, hand and wrist and I can step slowly, carefully guarding my balance.

I am now wearing a different brace on my arm and hand, one that seems to be encouraging my hand to hold itself open in a more natural position. My therapist calls it a resting hand splint. I had been holding it in a painful, clenched position since the earlier days after my stroke. Now it is such a relief to see my fingers open and to even respond to signals from my brain.

One day at a time, as they say.

CHAPTER 2:   A BRAIN TEASER

Please understand that because of my brain injury, I am concentrating ever intensely in order to assemble my thoughts as I move through each paragraph of this text. While my thoughts eventually do come together, it sometimes takes a little longer than it would other people. I am finding it very therapeutic to attempt to assemble each paragraph for this book and I hope you are able to do the same if you ever take on the challenge of putting your stroke or any such experience in writing.

You must remember that having the confidence to put the details of a traumatic event down in writing can be very therapeutic, not to mention extremely interesting. I hope you are able to do this. Please also remember that the purpose of this exercise is to stimulate the brain and that you should feel a sense of accomplishment in doing so. You should not feel overwhelmed by this, as is likely because you are using your brain at what may seem like an overwhelming pace. I can tell you from experience that it is like being in a different world with the pressure in your head telling you to stop or slow down.

I would think that you probably should have your neurologist's support before undertaking any such project. I am certainly not particularly qualified to comment on this one way or the other. I am simply a determined stroke survivor, living one day at a time, in the hopes of one day regaining some semblance of my former life.

CHAPTER 3:   A POSITIVE ATTITUDE

There is nothing more important than to have a positive attitude and to take an aggressive approach to coping with a sickness, particularly one as serious as stroke. It becomes ever so important to take control of your life. Most of us probably never had to worry about our health until such time as a catastrophe such as this strikes, and now it is our foremost responsibility to get tough and tackle the challenge.

A stroke survivor's life will have changed drastically and by now will have become a war. To succeed you must be strong. It is up to you. So many times, you will hear a patient say that they trust their doctor. While desirable, unfortunately, he or she is not going to be there with you all day, each and every day. Your doctor is only one component of your battle against your plight. This battle will require you to take the initiative at every opportunity and to persevere.

Recently, I had some business cards printed up with the following inscription:

A STROKE SURVIVOR
LIVING A DIFFERENT LIFE, FOR NOW
SEE YOU ON THE COURTS OR ON THE GREEN!

I am attempting to persevere with some of the activities I enjoyed prior to my stroke, including tennis and golf. My goal is clear; my attitude, my determination, Taoist Tai Chi, physiotherapy, continued exercise, acupuncture and TCM (traditional Chinese medicine) will help me reach it.

CHAPTER 4: BECOME INFORMED

Please understand that, in this story, I am attempting to recall my personal nightmare as accurately and as clearly as possible for the benefit of others who may also be going through a similar maze of pain, with its many confusing thoughts and ongoing challenges. As I try to express the details of my experience, it is reasonable to expect tears of emotion to occasionally well up and dominate my efforts to overcome the discomfort. These feelings should be natural for people with normal skills and abilities. This story is intended to provide some idea or understanding of what people who have had a stroke like this are going through, because I am certainly finding that many people have no idea what this experience is like, nor do they have any idea what this isolated world could possibly feel like.

Once a disease or illness as serious as cancer or stroke enters your life, you must become as knowledgeable about your condition as humanly possible. In fact, it actually becomes a full-time job that will last as long as the sickness or affliction itself. Many patients assume that they don't need any knowledge or experience since they have an "excellent" doctor or are getting the required care. But there are many times when your specific and pertinent knowledge will become invaluable.

It will also be necessary to become involved in making decisions on the various types of treatment available to you, as well as the different and ever-changing medications you can be prescribed. Evaluating the doctor's comments and advice on your medicine, your immune system and your diet is a fundamental part of defeating or overcoming such illnesses. You don't want to duck a responsibility that seems to lie only with the doctor.

A cancer or stroke support group can be a great source of knowledge and encouragement. You should try to join a good group that provides information, commonality and companionship, not just sympathy. Exchanging ideas and experiences with other people who are walking or have walked in your shoes will give you not only valuable insight but will, in many cases, give you hope that things will improve, even though it may seem like a long, slow process.

For example, I recently met a woman who is a travel consultant at a local agency that specializes in cruises. Kim also had a stroke, eight years ago, but you would never know it! Like me, she was working in an extremely stressful job, commuting long distances and raising two young children with her equally busy husband. One day, she simply collapsed. While you would never know anything about her previous crisis to look at her, she told me that, to this day, she still has an area on her left cheek that feels as though it has been injected with Novocain. She also said that her left arm feels as though it was someone else's and was sewn onto her. There is no feeling whatsoever, although she has full use of it.

Anyway, I guess my purpose in mentioning Kim here is that I found her to be an inspiration and that speaking with her and seeing her walking around as though nothing ever happened to her gave me hope. So, you see, there is light at the end of the tunnel! Meeting people like this is what helps keep me going when I start feeling sorry for myself which, let's face it, we are all inclined and are entitled to do once in a while! My thanks and admiration are due to Kim, Andy, Drew, Kelly, Mary and Bernice and all my Taoist Tai Chi instructors, assistant instructors and co-participants for all their help, inspiration and encouragement. Thank you, Thank you, Thank you, Thank you! I shall be eternally grateful.

CHAPTER 5: DON'T SWEAT THE SMALL STUFF

Thanks to my Tai Chi friend and co-participant, Andy, I have been able to make subtle yet meaningful adjustments to my overall outlook on life. Andy has taught me that when you have become stricken with a serious illness or have a debilitating accident, you may discover that your co-workers and those who you thought were your close friends and even sometimes your family will often forget about you or start to pay very little attention to you. If this happens, you need to do yourself a favour and just forget about it. Put it all behind you and just don't dwell on it. Most people have their own problems and issues to deal with. Their lives aren't necessarily in as much order as you would normally expect. You shouldn't worry about things or situations you just can't seem to be able to control or change.

If there's one thing I've learned through this whole experience, it is that life is short and we owe it to ourselves to take full advantage of every moment. Carpe diem! Seize the day! I've also learned to choose my battles. The little things just aren't worth hassling over.

"Don't sweat the small stuff!", as Andy would say.

EPILOGUE

Well, as you can see, I am alive today. I am still hopeful for a satisfactory recovery. I have some brain damage that affects my short-term memory and restricts my ability to move my leg, arm and hand the way they are supposed to. So far, I can't play my guitar. I am, however, participating in some sports activities. I am enjoying myself in my new life.

How can there be unfaltering faith when life can be so drastically altered from what it used to be? Hélène has discouraged me from being so harsh about these Christian issues so I am backing off from them just a little. However, as an author, albeit a new and fairly inexperienced one, I am determined to tell it like it is. Hélène has easily convinced me that we are rich in love with each other and we are lucky with that and the boys and Cooper, our wonderful Golden Retriever. I suppose I am happy and lucky to be able to get on with a very different life and I have entertained myself with writing this book and know that we will plan some very special holidays together in years ahead. As each week goes by, Hélène and I remind each other of how much we love each other and how lucky we are. Each day, we are hopeful that I will have more recovery. Although there are no guarantees that much of my misfortune isn't permanent, I continue my physiotherapy with as much determination as I can muster and I will continue to track and document every development as I continue to recover. My progress to date has been capably managed by my various physiotherapists, who I appreciate so much and can't thank enough for their relentless efforts in pushing me forward.

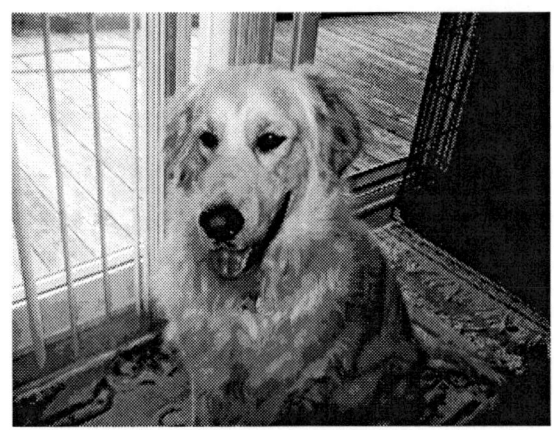

Cooper, ca. 2005

My life so far has been an incredible journey. I am not famous, nor have I done anything significant for the world…yet. I lost two good friends during my adolescence. I lost the best friend a man could ask for about six years ago. I was honored to be able to deliver a eulogy that I never would have thought I would be placed in a position to do. I once jumped off a swinging pedestrian bridge over a rushing river and never hurt myself because I judged and knew exactly what I was doing…entertaining my friends!

As you might imagine and can possibly detect, I am an angry, but somewhat 'with it', stroke survivor. The daily and ongoing pain and discomfort I seem to endure are sometimes almost unbearable and the constant pressure and traffic in my head creates confusion about nearly everything I have to process and think about. I have always been a rather intensely focused individual where I usually seem to have so much on my mind. Now, since my stroke, I think I am probably doing myself a disservice by allowing and encouraging too many thoughts and issues to continually saturate my neurological well-being.

At this time, I am continuing to practice Taoist Tai Chi and occasionally go to physiotherapy. I am walking with a cane and a brace. I have recently learned about meditation in my Taoist Tai Chi Health Recovery classes and I feel that I am beginning to learn about how to take control of and stabilize my mental and cognitive state. While I am sitting here, writing away, I am reflecting on my situation, occasionally chatting with my wife or any of my sons. My thoughts are saturated with the internal and ongoing summarizing I constantly do of my new life: unable to walk, play guitar or participate in many of the sports and activities that I used to enjoy. Yes, but in some ways, I am lucky and am still hanging on to some of the things I used to do. Things like playing tennis and golf, which I am currently still actively including in my drastically modified and compromised life.

I still need to make a very important statement here. If you have the slightest suspicion that symptoms of stroke exist, get your butt to your doctor and make sure you educate yourself regarding all issues pertaining to stroke. A good book to read is "Stroke, A Comprehensive Guide to Brain Attacks". And make sure you read and understand it all! And follow up and take it seriously! If you have the slightest hint of any of the symptoms, do something about it! You do have a problem that needs to be fixed. They left me out of the process. No one slapped me in the face and told me to smarten up! I had been healthy all my life. I never paid too much attention to my family physician's diagnosis of high blood pressure where he had simply put me on a prescription of Cozar initially, then Hyzar. He then prescribed Norvasc in addition to the Hyzar. In this type of situation, the doctor needs to grab you firmly by the shoulders, look right into your eyes and say: "Look, you g@# d@#n f**ing idiot, if you don't take your medicine religiously, get an at-home blood pressure monitor and watch your b.p. closely, lose some weight, get more exercise, watch your alcohol intake or if you experience headaches (which I never used to), you'd best get your ass in to a hospital lickety split!"

I had gone to the hospital and was checked over, with the doctors identifying fairly high blood pressure, but I was just sent home with instructions to see my family doctor before the end of the week, which I did. Actually, throughout these visits, someone should have read me the Riot Act or even simply admitted me to hospital right then and there. But this is now history and I am now handicapped and living a different life with a modified plan of hopes and dreams. I am just lucky that I still have my family and the love and support that anyone would be so lucky to have. And life goes on.

Thank you for reading Stroke: A Long, Challenging Journey. I hope you have enjoyed reading it as much as I enjoyed writing it and sharing my new and former life and adventures with you. I hope this book is helpful and I want to apologize for any errors or misconceptions that may have occurred. My intentions and objectives were well-meaning. I have written this book for all my friends, loved ones and anyone else who may possibly read it and be able to benefit from it. Remember, earlier I said that I would play the guitar again (even if it just means you and I together, Bob). Therefore, there will be a sequel to this book.

I love my wife, my family and my incredibly altered and compromised life. I wish you all the best and good luck.

Love to you all!

pf

"Don't let the hardship from the past rob the joy from the present."

Author Unknown

IN CLOSING

Peter Frost is a pseudonym.

I have used only first names in these stories to ensure privacy. I will be sending publishing and distribution information to friends and loved ones in order to direct anyone who is interested to my book. If you know of or encounter anyone else who may also benefit from or who may possibly enjoy this book, please tell them about it and forward the title and ISBN # to them.

Please look for additional works by Peter Frost. I am currently working on my next book.

Also, I hope you enjoy the movie!

Peter

APPENDIX

A STROKE SURVIVOR'S JOURNAL - HOW I FEEL

In this section, I will attempt to describe for you just how I am feeling on a day-to-day basis, to provide some understanding of what I am going through and a bit of what is happening inside my head each day. Besides sharing this information, my objective here is to reassure and encourage other stroke survivors that whatever they are experiencing is not unique, nor is it uncharacteristic of this tragedy called "stroke". I can't be too sure that these feelings and experiences are the same for every stroke survivor but let me tell you that, from every conversation I have had with other stroke survivors, we all are pretty much feeling many of the same symptoms, depending on the severity of our respective strokes. For example, in my case, I had two hemorrhagic bleeds which have left me with total paralysis on my left side. I have little or no use of my left limbs and I endure numbness and a "frozen" feeling on the left side of my face. I cannot feel or use my left hand, arm, leg or foot and I constantly have excruciating pain (thalamic pain/CPS) in the extremities of my left side.

Considering I am experiencing all of these symptoms on a daily basis, I feel as though I have walked miles towards a recovery that still seems so far down the road. But I have to persevere and so must all of you! Or if you are smart and have not traveled this route already, you will let these recollections scare the %#&@ out of you and you will take appropriate care of yourself and have your blood pressure checked.

To give you an idea of what I go through on a daily basis, I have included the following logs from my journal. I hope that reading them will encourage and reassure readers if they are experiencing anything resembling what I have gone and am still going through. It is my hope that sharing these experiences with others will help make them aware that they are not alone and will help them through their own journey.

I started this log in March, 2005 to help me follow and understand what it was I was going through. I continued it reasonably faithfully until March, 2006 and now make only the occasional entry. I began writing this book in March, 2005 and it is now July, 2006. I am just in the final stages of completing it. I have written over 100,000 words and have printed three rough copies of 250 to 300 8 ½" x 11" pages.

Hélène and I are just now feverishly attempting to apply the finishing touches to the last bits of the final chapters. I have pretty much completed most of the content and my wonderful wife has been committing much time to editing and typing many of the corrections that I have scribbled over words and entered in the margins. We both have fairly astute spelling and grammar skills and so we believe that our editing should have been sufficient for this first-time author-works. Every time I think I am just about done, I think of something else I want or need to write about. For example, recently I was admitted to a rehab program at the Whitby Day Hospital. So now I have another wonderful chapter of this **long, challenging journey** to write, entitled **REHABILITATION**. My physiatrist actually referred me to this facility the last time I saw him. It is an amazing place with some incredible people!

You can read about it in Section 5, Chapter 7.

March 24, 2005

Today, I feel quite lethargic; I am short of breath; I feel cold and clammy. I also feel like I have diarrhea, or at the very least like I need to go to the bathroom all the time. My teeth hurt. I have a slight headache. My blood pressure is normal. My lips feel numb and my left foot feels frozen, although it is warm to the touch. I also feel extremely dizzy, which is the new normal for me. I have difficulty focusing and concentrating. It feels good to just go to sleep and forget everything.

I have reported these issues to my doctors in the past, but nothing I complain about ever seems too alarming. I am usually told that only time will relieve some of these symptoms. Still, I just feel that things are not that right and I want a pill or to be given an operation or some medical procedure to end this. I am so fed up!

March 30, 2005

From one day to the next, I never know how I'm going to feel. Some days are not too bad; I can be cheerful, energetic and almost "normal". Then, the next day, for some unexplained reason, I feel lethargic, I ache all over, particularly my extremities and my breathing is shallow. I just want to sleep it all away.

Hélène and I have discovered that taking it easy and keeping my head calm seems to help me get through the discomfort. Case in point: last Christmas, Hélène gave me tickets to the Eagles' concert at the Air Canada Centre in Toronto. I was so excited! This is a band I have loved and admired for many years. I had seen them once before (in

Ottawa actually) and Hélène had never seen them. As the concert day approached, we were both really pumped.

Unfortunately, for about a week or so prior to the concert date, I was feeling particularly uncomfortable and was experiencing considerable pain (everywhere, not any particular location). I also had an earache, although two doctors had indicated that there was no evidence of any infection. My breathing was labored and I was very lethargic, to the point of having to miss my physiotherapy and occupational therapy two days in a row. I was seriously beginning to think I wouldn't be well enough to make the trip downtown. Somehow, my determination got us there anyway.

Yesterday morning (the day of the concert), I woke up feeling not too bad but still unsure of how I would be feeling at the end of the day. Hélène and I discussed it and decided that the best thing for me to do was to lay low all day so I would hopefully have the energy to travel on the commuter train at 5 o'clock. As it turned out, we were right. I was feeling much better by the time we were ready to leave for the train and the entire evening was a huge success. Obviously, conserving my energy that day was the right thing to do! Hélène and I are sitting here at the keyboard this very moment reflecting on the wonderful Christmas present she gave me.

Actually, as we are sitting here, we are both feeling a little sore. For me, it's my left hand that is aching. In Hélène's case, it's both her hands and her wrists as she suffers from arthritis. Well, I must share with you this fabulous new product we came across recently – a wonder drug, in my opinion – called 024. It is an essential oil pain neutralizer that consists of camphor, eucalyptus, menthol and aloe vera. Hélène rubbed some on both my hand and hers and we were both pain-free five minutes later! It is incredible and is available over the counter to anyone who needs it.

April 4, 2005

Well, by comparison, I'm feeling not too bad today but I didn't get around to writing down how I actually felt yesterday. I sort of remember that it was not that great a day, but today is definitely a better day. As I've said before, from one day to the next, I never really know just how I'm going to feel but today, I'm feeling pretty good, almost normal but just with the usual tightness in my leg, arm, hand and fingers. Unfortunately, I'm never feeling absolutely normal or totally comfortable anymore because I'm afraid that isn't quite yet attainable with the brain damage that I have experienced. I have just had a shower and am now sitting quietly at my computer and I am not encountering any of the potential pain I can usually expect to be afflicted by on any given day; however, my head continues to ring as it always does but is allowing me to complete some thoughts on the PC and get some work done on this book. To try to describe as accurately as possible how my head feels and likely how most other similarly brain damaged people are feeling, it is as though my skull feels like 2,000 little 'sons of bitches' have been running around inside my head with 4lb rubber mallets, swinging away like crazy, doing whatever additional damage they can do. Another way I have learned to describe it is as though someone has taken the top off of my skull and is swishing away inside it with an egg beater. This sensation inside my head is not quite painful, but it feels like a door buzzer has been wired with a low voltage electric current inside my head. With the charge is a severe numbing sensation that starts at the base of my neck and creeps up the back of my skull, feeling like the skin at the beginning of my scalp has been folded and squeezed together tightly with pliers. Also, what I am trying to say is how inescapable this always is.

So, today, I am much more comfortable with only a bit of the usual dizziness that drives me so friggin' nuts. Phew!

April 6, 2005

Beginning part way through the morning, before taking my meds, I was feeling pretty much the same as yesterday, which is extremely dizzy, with intense pressure at the back of my head and poor concentration and balance. I also, once again, have extreme tightness at the back of my head and a burning sensation in my fingers as though I am being stung by 100 bees.

I have a moderate headache and am experiencing some (borderline) queasiness in my stomach. I am very lethargic and I just want to go to sleep.

Now that I've had my meds, I'm still pretty lethargic but not necessarily as dizzy.

April 7, 2005

Amazingly enough, for most of today, I have actually not been feeling too bad. Sometimes, I feel lethargic and my head feels congested and slow to react.

When I began the day, I was actually feeling pretty normal, even perky and fairly responsive. I left the house at about 10:45 this morning to begin my routine of physio at

Ajax-Pickering Hospital at 11:00 am, lunch at the hospital, occupational therapy at 1:00 pm. I went through my physio drills without a problem and had a nice lunch in the hospital cafeteria with Hélène.

After occupational therapy, we left the hospital and went on a major shopping trip to Home Depot, etc. and I still continued to feel pretty good, even joking around with the staff at Home Depot. When I got home, I laid down before dinner. Now, it is 8:30 pm or so and I am not feeling the pains or tingling in my toes or my fingers as is customary, but I am a little lethargic and feeling dizzy and not concentrating or thinking too well at the moment. It is almost as though I get used to these feelings from one moment to another.

April 9, 2005

I can tell this is not going to be one of my greatest days. My left side is not feeling too great (stinging and tingling). There are days when I can't really complain but, at the moment, I am feeling a little thick headed, which means I need to turn my head slowly because my neck is stiff. My head is buzzing, particularly around my left ear which aches terribly. Unfortunately, Tylenol never seems to help. I have complained about this and have been to the doctor and the hospital about it but there is never any sign of an infection and apparently nothing can be done. Cripes, I just want to get up and walk this all off and pretend it is all a bad dream, but I guess that's another life, hopefully down the road! Also, the nerve endings in my left fingers and toes are tingling painfully. Again, I try to remain positive about the possibility that this is an indication that some feeling is returning to some of my extremities, but it sure is painful and to have what I describe as "the little sons of bitches inside my head, swinging 4lb rubber mallets" sure drives me friggin' nuts though!

At the moment, I am on the verge of a nasty headache but I think I am well enough to go out to the Great Canadian Superstore and shop for groceries with my wife. Gee, I love that store; we are always a little hungry when we go there and we buy a plate of raw vegetables and dip for a mid-day snack. Amazingly enough, for most of today, I have actually been feeling not too bad. Sometimes I feel lethargic and my head feels congested and slow to react. Other times, I feel as though my head is going to clear and I will wake up feeling normal again.

April 10, 2005

This is another crappy day when my head feels like it wants to explode. Today, I guess I spent too much time on the PC and it has congested my head. I think I have figured out that too much reading and PC use and the associated concentration is one of the main contributing patterns to this friggin' dizziness! Maybe it happens when I am concentrating on too many other things, too or when things frustrate or disappoint me. I will call it traffic! I will continue to write such patterns down and look for possible remedies. No doctor as yet has offered this as a likely cause but I will be ecstatic if someone tells me that this all makes sense, is normal, is predictable and will get better one day. I am closely monitoring these things and think that this makes perfect sense from what I have observed. Actually, my head is so dizzy right now and feels like it is bound tightly with an elastic band. I just want to roll my eyes back and sleep all the time. When I feel this way, sleeping is such a relief because everything that is bothering me goes away. My toes are okay today, just the balls of my feet are tingling and I feel lethargic. So all in all, it is looking like a better day!

April 11, 2005

Once again, I guess I spent too much time on the PC and reading and my head is once more feeling very congested. I find that some friends I have gotten to know who have similar brain problems experience the same frustration in trying to get answers, explanations or fixes (my research has led me to understand that this pain is called Thalamic Pain) and have similar difficulties and experiences with their head. I am closely monitoring these things and writing details down each day so that, in the event there is a pattern, it will help me understand what's going on and maybe others can identify similar feelings.

April 12, 2005

I am not feeling as dizzy today as I was yesterday, however my left hand is tingling again and is extremely painful. This has improved by the end of the day. I have a slight headache and I am feeling lethargic and my head is numb. My lips also are numb, as though they have been injected with Novocain or I have been punched squarely in the mouth. My abdominal area is tingling and vibrating. I talk with a hoarse voice and I'm short of breath as I speak. I feel a bit better than I did yesterday but I am very sick and tired of feeling so shitty almost every day, unable to do anything about it or even to take a pill to make it all go away. Hélène and Cooper and I went for a walk today then I did some of my stretching exercises after we came in. The air was cool, fresh and invigorating. I am feeling not too badly at the moment and it seems as though today may eventually end up being a better day than yesterday. I'll wait and see how I feel later.

Over the past few days, I have been feeling pretty crappy. My head is still ringing most of the time. It has become important to my well-being and my mood to write down how I feel each day because, with my memory loss, I don't recall how or what I was feeling from one day to the next. I just feel the impulse to have more control over this feeling. Please understand that I did not intend to offend anyone by what I said a few paragraphs earlier about my frustration in not finding a solution to this problem. In my efforts to write about this nightmare and share my experience, I just want to scream out loud about how I feel. More than anything, I want to get better. Hopefully, through this experience I will help others improve their situation as well. You can't imagine the lost, desperate feeling. Then again, I know that some of you do understand and I wish you good luck also in your personal quests.

April 13, 2005

Today has the promise of being a better day. I am tired and am lying down after my shower. My dizziness is not too bad so far today. I will stay away from the computer today (this morning anyway!) and may not even attempt to get back to it until tonight. I've been logging how I feel each day and I may just stop so that I can get on with other things that are on my mind. Hélène and I are so busy just trying to get our papers in order in preparation for filing our 2004 income tax returns. I did some shredding of old files this morning and Hélène has done all the filing (months of it!).

April 18, 2005

Today we drove to Renfrew to visit my dad, my sister and my niece. It is a four hour drive with a couple of stops. While we were driving along the 401, I started to feel a bizarre, fine, popping sensation like kids' "pop rocks" candy bursting in my head. When the sensation finally stopped a few moments later, the customary dizziness in my head had gone! What a wonderful relief! My head felt unbelievably clear. Unfortunately, this unusual feeling did not last for more than about 25 minutes! At this point, there is no explanation for this that we understand. We have never heard of such an occurrence, despite all the exposure to stroke-related issues to which we have been privy. This phenomenon gives me hope that some day this dizziness will eventually go away! You can be sure we will be talking to my Neurologist about this one!

I felt better for only about 25 minutes and then the dizziness started to gradually come back. Soon I was back to my former sick self and felt lousy again for the rest of the day and into the evening when we met up in a pub with some good friends I used to hang around with back in the early 1970s. We spent a few hours reminiscing over some unbelievably good times and wild adventures that we all somehow fortunately survived. It almost seemed like the stimulation of the conversation and laughs with them made my head dizzier, making me feel awful again. The friends included Garry, his wife Karen,

John, his wife Laurie, Donnie and his wife Donna. The only one missing from this band of good old buddies was Gerard, who was at home in Ottawa.

That night, I didn't sleep well. I'm not sure if it was because of the extra stimulation (or traffic!) or the fact that I was sleeping in a strange bed in a hotel, but I was uncomfortable and in pain all night.

April 19, 2005

Today my head feels like it's going to split open, no exaggeration! Most days, my head feels very congested. I just want to scream and shake it until whatever might be crammed in there crumbles and falls out through my left ear, which aches so bad. My left ear often feels as though it is infected and needs to be treated with Amoxicillin or some other antibiotic. The bizarre thing is that at another moment, the dizziness subsides, the ear ache goes away and I don't even remember how badly I felt.

However, since I have been analyzing how I feel each day and writing down how each area of my body is feeling, I can compare it to other days when I have felt better. I have come to the conclusion that my head exponentially worsens whenever I increase the volume of traffic that I am attempting to process at the time. Sometimes too much social interaction has the same awful effect.

Also, I have decided that the best way to describe the feeling inside my head is to compare it to what it might be like standing in the middle of the road at the intersection of Highways 401 and 404 (probably the busiest intersection in North America) on a long holiday weekend, standing there on rollerblades, being precariously and viciously spun around as north, south, east and westbound traffic relentlessly whizzes by in all directions. Augh!!

For example, if I am working on the computer (and remember, I have written 10,000 or so more words towards my book in the past few weeks) and put deep thought into whatever I am writing at the moment or if I am thinking about what I am going through, the dizziness increases, the pressure in my head becomes intolerable and I just want to sleep. I am told that there is no pill for this, that only time can possibly heal whatever is going on inside my brain. The major part of the discomfort is the pressure and tightness towards the back of my neck and up to the inside of my skull.

May 20, 2005

To top everything off, I am now experiencing my fourth bladder infection since I was discharged from my initial rehab program at Bridgepoint Health a year and a half ago. If you have ever had a bladder infection, you know what I mean when I say "I just want to die!" Not only is this not fun, but it is, without any doubt, the worst feeling you can imagine. You become lethargic and the 'head rushes' just don't stop.

Although I was diagnosed with yet another bladder infection, I am pleased to say this week has not been the worst. After conducting a urine test the other day, my physician has told me of the presence of yet another bladder infection which has gotten me scared of what's to come as I can't help but remember how poorly I felt during the last one.

I already have fairly severe dizziness as a result of my brain surgery, but, compounded with the effects of another urinary tract infection, I simply cannot think straight nor do I even want or feel able to hold my head up. The back of my neck hurts; I have a slight headache and I am quite lethargic. I want so badly to be able to express how I feel today yet all I want to do is go to bed and sleep for a year! I actually look forward to swallowing the however many pills I take twice a day in the hopes that they will soon rid my body of the obvious poisons.

For each of the last three times I have had a bladder infection, and this time as well, I have more than anxiously awaited the end of this torture. I have become so accustomed to this feeling that I can actually practically predict the onset of another bout of this painful infection.

May 22, 2005

I have woken early, as usual, and feel good so far except for a stiff neck and a burning sensation in my toes. I have come to regard this as not too bad a start to the day. My wife also has just gotten up, given me a nice wet kiss, is running herself a bath and has gotten me a cold glass of cranberry juice. The day looks promising! Cooper is playing tug-of-war with me with his rubber toy and I'm promising myself and my wife to not do too much whining today. It probably should be a pretty good day. I have just had my shower by my homecare worker and am refreshed and ready to take on the day! Only a minor head buzz is happening so far as I speak!

May 27, 2005

It is Friday morning and, once more, I am not feeling well. I could sense this coming on because I have been experiencing the typical symptoms of yet another bladder infection creeping on. I have just finished the prescribed medication for seven days for the last urinary tract infection and have a requisition for another urine test to make sure my body is clear of it. I have gotten to know the pattern of the onset of the infection and I know I can't count on one day of feeling better to let me know or tell me I'm okay. Unless I have an all-clear from a urine test, I just know the infection will be ravaging my body and my head again in no time. When I have one of these infections, I become extremely dizzy, get lethargic and have to pee frequently. I also experience double vision and become so dizzy that my eyes can't focus or adjust. Fortunately through all this grief, I usually never feel nauseous or get headaches. I would trade this feeling for anything however. I almost wish the medical experts could try this feeling on for size so that we, the patients, could be sure they knew what this illness feels like and they could be focusing on developing an accurate treatment and cure. I never feel as though I am being taken seriously or being closely listened to. As I said, one feeling seems to blend into the other.

May 28, 2005

This is going to be a so-so day, but not one of my worst. I can sense the onset of one of my ongoing bladder infections. I am very obstinate and insistent with Hélène that I will not feel comfortable or confident that this curse is gone unless I have another urine test and have absolute confirmation that the infection is gone. I am so uncertain of whether the bladder infection is restarting its gradual rampage or if I am just about to have another ongoing head rush from my brain damage.

One symptom just seems to flow into the other. My bladder infection pattern has become so familiar. I feel as though it seems to be trying to take over again. I also have extreme tingling in my fingers again. It feels like 1,000 bee stings, no exaggeration. I also think that I am figuring out that it is the exercises and stretching that I do to the joints and tendons a few times a day that are causing this discomfort. It seems that the stinging feeling blends in with the paralysis of my left hand and before I actually realize it, I am in constant and deep-rooted pain which eventually goes away and is nearly totally gone the next day. This concerns me because my fingers are very stiff and become locked and I want to continue to stretch and exercise them. I am afraid that I could be doing damage but I want so much to unlock them and open them and try to get them close to being back to normal. My physiotherapist just says the tingling and stinging feeling 'is bad!' I want to have an x-ray and get a definitive prognosis so that I can know if I can continue to stretch them. I wonder if I am being unreasonable. I don't know. I'm no f'n specialist. I just want to get better.

As I sit here at the PC, having just written this section, I am just realizing that I am not feeling as badly as I have been in recent weeks. Geez, I actually think I am going to have a better day. I am a bit dizzy however, but we have tentative plans to do a lot of things this weekend. Today, if it isn't raining, we are going to Camp X, a military historical exhibit; tomorrow, we're going to a Golden Retriever rescue BBQ with other friends. We are also having them back to the house for beer and snacks afterward. All of this, of course, will depend on the weather.

May 29, 2005

Well, by the time we got home last night (after seeing the new Star Wars movie), I was once again feeling absolutely awful. I kept having the urge to pee, but only a few drops came each time. I was also experiencing a burning sensation down my left side. All in all, not a good feeling!

This morning, I woke up at about 6:00 am and started doing some work on the PC. By the time Hélène got up, I was feeling like this was not going to be a good day. Once more, I have this overwhelming feeling that I've got yet another bladder infection. I'm so furious! What is it going to take to get this out of my system? I've been on antibiotics twice in the past three weeks, for God's sake. Enough, already!

Anyway, I'm taking it easy this afternoon, having decided that I wasn't feeling well enough to go to the Golden Retriever picnic today. Too bad. It would've been fun to see Cooper romping with all those other Goldens. Hopefully we can do it next year.

Right now, I have a burning sensation inside my left wrist, on top of my left hand and on my left index finger as well. Also, my face is numb (particularly my lips) and I just feel as though I want to sleep. My breathing is shallow and I feel a fine vibration (sort of shivering, fine tremor type of feeling) in my chest and stomach. I have tingling in both ears, but mostly my left ear, which feels like an earache. My left arm is very stiff, feeling like it is pulling up and into my left side, a little like being elbowed in the lower part of my rib cage. I am not feeling very comfortable with all these different sensations happening all the time. The tightness in my head at the back of my neck is the most uncomfortable. It almost feels as though someone has sliced me up the middle of the back of my neck. It makes it difficult for me to think or concentrate and my vision is blurry.

The urge to pee comes and goes all day and I am cold and clammy much of the time. At times, these sensations seem to overwhelm me and I just want to cry. I can certainly sense yet another bladder infection (U.T.I.) coming on.

May 30, 2005

Today, I feel discomfort on my left side that I would compare to someone digging their elbow into my side. It's not really painful, just terribly uncomfortable. Earlier this morning, I was up working on my PC at 6:00 am, back to bed at 8:30 or so and then back to sleep until 11:30 am. I guess I was tired! I was given a shower by my PSW early this afternoon and felt quite lethargic afterwards, so I lay down and had a snooze for part of the afternoon.

At 4:00 pm my personal trainer, Angie, came in and put me through my paces. Man, does it ever feel good whenever she stretches my limbs! My whole body feels invigorated afterward. My left leg is extremely stiff today and my left knee is cracking a lot, which isn't necessarily unusual and there seems to be quite a bit of resistance in my leg as Angie takes me through my stretches. We have also noticed that my left foot seems somewhat swollen although I remember it as the normal shape of my foot which is due to my fallen arches. Or it could simply be because I tend to turn my left foot outwards when I walk.

May 31, 2005

So far today, I feel pretty good except for the usual unrelenting, severe dizziness that never goes away for a moment. I have gotten so used to it that I just tend to try to work through the discomfort. As I sit here at my PC this afternoon, I am swaying and my head is buzzing BIG TIME. And guess what? My family doctor's office has just called and said that, sure enough, I have another f'n bladder infection, exactly as I had predicted. I had sent in a urine test a few days back, Thursday night I guess it was. I was told to wait until Tuesday for the results of the test, was not given medication to start treatment and Bingo! Here I am on Tuesday afternoon, told that I certainly do have another bladder infection. I am once more being given a prescription of 'Macrobid' which was not effective the last time and must start another 7 day/twice a day dose of the antibiotic but I have lost the momentum of the first dose. So once more I am starting to feel lethargic, have acute dizziness and slight pains in my lower rib cage area. I find it difficult to sit up straight and concentrate. I am experiencing a slight numbness in my lips. If the pattern remains the same as each other time this sickness has overcome me, I should be feeling terrible within the next 24 hours. We are awaiting the medication prescription to be faxed to the pharmacy so that we can go and get the pills. I have my Lear Jet on the ready to go and get the prescription as soon as it is ready. In fact, the fax has just been sent, Hélène has picked up the pills, and I have taken my first of 14 more pills. Here we go again!

June 8, 2005

The tingling in my fingers and toes and the numbness that is occurring inside my head are so intense that I do not ever recall feeling this way three or four months ago. I have never gotten an explanation for what exactly this is or why it is happening or even if it is a bad thing. It is worse now than it ever was. Am I simply healing? Is this a good thing? Oh, I think I am being told that it is just nerve endings repairing themselves. So, I suppose it is a good thing. Well, small graces!

It is happening in my head and my neck mostly. I feel as though I am straining my neck all the time. It is a strain on my eyes. I feel a pressure on the left side of my head and I feel a tingling in my left hand and wrist.

June 11, 2005

A typical day for me these days usually begins by opening my eyes, I suppose not unlike anyone else! However for me and, I suppose, any other stroke survivor who has had a similar brain affliction, I wake up only to begin a very familiar pattern. I usually slowly regain consciousness from a peaceful sleep. Before my stroke, I used to always have a sound, uninterrupted sleep and woke perfectly rested, ready to start a new, interesting and adventurous day. Sometimes that consisted of a typical full, busy day at work or it might be a day off, either because it was a holiday, some well-earned vacation time or maybe was just the weekend. No matter what, I always woke up feeling rested. Now, I can honestly say that even with my 24/7 fierce brain buzz, I fortunately still usually get a good night's sleep. Sometimes I do seem to take a while to fall asleep so I turn on the TV and watch a bit of a good WWII DVD or perhaps a documentary that happens to be on at that time. This is simply one of my most favorite things to do, because of my Dad's successful and exciting involvement in the war. Or I might read a bit of a good book if I happen to have one on the go. Of course, during the lengthy period I have been working on my book, I usually scribble some notes into my handy notebook beside the bed (quietly so as not to disturb or wake Hélène). I haven't been reading much since I had my stroke because my vision can be a bit blurry and I sometimes find it difficult to focus and concentrate. I pick up a book to read and actually get through anywhere from five to ten pages, put the book down for a refreshment or whatever and totally forget about the book I was reading and never pick it up again. So I have five books on the go right now that I started with the best of intentions but never get around to picking up again. The same goes for audio books. I currently have two of those on the go. I find all this very frustrating. Here I am with all kinds of time (?) for reading, yet I never seem to get around to resuming any one of them!

Anyway, whatever the time, I say good morning to my sweetie, parking a wet kiss on her lips and jump up and slide out of bed, and I am instantly ready to start my day.

June 26, 2005

The last few days have been incredible and actually just an unbelievable experience in my recovery efforts. These past few days have given me hope, encouragement and inspiration. It all started on Wednesday, June 22. It was an incredibly hot day, as it had been for the past few days and was forecasted for the next week or so. We had gotten off to a great start for the summer with some beautiful weather and we were looking forward to and had started to enjoy many days in our 16' x 32' above ground pool.

So on Wednesday, Angie, my personal trainer came over and she and Hélène and I had gotten into the pool to enjoy a refreshing dip and do some leg-strengthening and some cardiovascular exercises. You must understand that getting into the pool is not exactly a straightforward exercise for us/me. Of course, I have the extreme paralysis on my left side and am not able to simply step down the moulded stairway we have installed to enter our 4' deep pool. I have very little dorsiflexion in my left foot and my left leg is totally stiff.

I have to approach the pool in my wheelchair and Hélène carefully gets my left foot down the first step. I must take the first step leading with my left foot, which, at one time, could not even bear any weight without considerable pain. I cannot flex my left foot at all, but I am able to carefully get it down with full weight to the first step, and then easily follow with my right foot so that I am comfortably standing on the first step, holding the rail firmly with my right hand. Remember, my left hand doesn't work, so balance and steadiness is always a challenge. I always lead with my left foot and then follow with my right. I repeat this for each of the subsequent four steps until I am firmly standing at the fourth or second last step, then Hélène lets go of me and I simply fall forward, holding my breath as I make a face first, full splash into the pool. I am successfully in the pool, pushing off in a dead man's float for about 8 or 10 feet while I slowly regroup and catch my breath and regain my composure.

Now, I can relax and forget the nervousness of the entry procedure. I am in and ready to float and push off with my right foot, my life jacket comfortably and securely in place. I have to tell you that this entry is always hard work for the two of us, with Hélène having to take my full weight a number of times as I progress down the stairs. It is a lot more straightforward when there are three of us with the third person able to help guide my foot as I go down the stairs. In fact, until recently, we never even attempted to get me in the water unless there was a third person there to help. Now, it can either be just the two of us or sometimes another person helping us and joining us for a swim.

Well, on this particular day, we were in the water and I began my routine of walking any amount of full laps to get my leg and foot warmed up and reasonably loose and into a pattern of stepping and pushing forward. I have to hold on to the pool rail with my right hand to hold myself up and enable me to break into a pattern of steps as I usually walk around the pool four or five times. I enjoy this gentle 0-weight exercise, feeling quite accomplished at each and every 96' lap. Remember, it is a 16' x 32' pool so the perimeter, and thus each lap, is 96'. I also have a routine of deep knee bends (Don Yus) which I had learned and was encouraged to do in my physiotherapy sessions and, of course, at my Tai Chi classes.

So, after a few Don Yus, I was lying on my back and I started kicking my legs. They were both moving equally and Angie, my personal trainer, suggested I try to do the same thing while lying on my stomach. She got me to flip over and, the next thing I knew, I was swimming across the pool! I went back and forth a half-dozen times or so and then decided to try to do the same thing lengthwise. So, I steadied myself at one end of the pool and began to topple forward. As my face approached the surface of the water and my feet pivoted on the bottom, I pushed off with my right foot, my left foot pretending to help. I lunged forward, body straight and began to body surf forward for the first couple of feet, totally relaxed, holding my breath and preparing to start taking the first strokes with my one good hand. My eyes were open, looking forward as I prepared to begin the natural motions of the front crawl, albeit with only half my functionality, using my good right arm and hand only and with the calm determination that I would pull and guide myself through the first 32' as smoothly as I was physically able.

By some unbelievable miracle, I realized that my hips were working pretty well (weren't paralyzed) and I could establish a routine of rhythmic kicking with both legs and I could straighten myself, holding my breath calmly and pulling and steering myself forward efficiently and accurately with my one good arm. So, I was able to swim the 32' from one end to the other with one breath and as I got to the end I simply stood up again, toppled forward once more and pushed off for yet another lap. My lungs were not strained, but Angie suggested I try to build in a "breath taking" at some point during the lap. I managed to do this and I proceeded to do ten complete laps successfully.

Since that day, every time I have gotten in the pool, I have added another lap to my goal. I am currently at 12 laps, non-stop, and who knows what I will be at in ten more days. I am extremely ecstatic and motivated by this accomplishment. Needless to say, Hélène is very proud of me and we have shared many hugs and kisses upon completion of each swim session.

June 28, 2005

Good Lord! Sure enough, I believe I have yet another bladder infection! No one has been able to explain exactly what this is I'm going through. All I know is that I want to scream! No, actually, it hurts so much, I just want to die. This is no normally tolerable feeling. My lips hurt. My paralyzed left arm is stinging so intensely. I have been told that any illness or infection such as this will tend to make stroke symptoms and the resulting pain more acute. The feeling in my arm and hand feels like 1,000 bee stings. I feel this for the most part right to the tips of my fingers and my toes, mostly my index finger and my middle finger, and in the palm of my hand. The inside of my wrist is entertaining 1,000 bee stings as well. I also have a similar sensation in my left foot, my left toes and up and down my left thigh and leg. My head aches and my neck hurts. This feeling is inescapable. I just want medicine, surgery or a cure!

I could tell that this bladder infection was coming on yesterday and I insisted and got a urine test in to my family doctor right away. Sure enough, the test came back positive. I wanted to scream!

My left ear hurts as does the left side of my face. I find it unusually frustrating that a person could feel this way without having to be rushed into the hospital for an operation of some sort. Apparently, this pain is either thalamic pain or regional pain and is quite normal in the stroke recovery process. Such pain usually starts to manifest itself approximately one year or so after the initial stroke.

I'm on the second day of the current infection's medication and I am desperately waiting for it to kick in. I take two tablets per day, 12 hours apart, one in the morning after breakfast and the other after supper. My throat is hoarse and I'm peeing all the time. I am very light-headed and my eyeballs ache and my eyes feel as though they're crossed, inverted in my head and staring upward with only the whites showing.

August 11, 2005

Having just returned home from a vacation trip by car to Ottawa, I am still feeling rather poorly like I started to feel during the fourth day of the seven day trip. My left arm and leg are very tight and stiff from my spasticity, and I am experiencing multiple spasms that hurt so very much. My face and neck also feel tight and painful. I have been moody and grouchy. I guess I was just feeling sorry for myself. I wish I could relax.

August 13, 2005

It is now two days since returning home from our little vacation in Ottawa to my own bed at home and I am feeling a little better but my hand is stinging. My head feels like a taught heavy gauge rubber band and my toes are stinging unbearably (feeling like 1,000 bee stings again). I am feeling a bit better today than the previous few days but I still find it difficult to concentrate or think straight. My index finger and big toe hurt the most.

Today, while surfing the internet, I was looking through some articles about spasticity and ITB (Intrathecal Baclofen) therapy for this problem. I came across an interesting and seemingly pertinent process of Baclofen-related therapy that appears to be beneficial for people with symptoms like mine. Please refer to this website for detailed information: www.medbroadcast.com, keyword *Baclofen*.

August 15, 2005

Today, as I was waking up, I was analyzing and trying to figure out how to best describe precisely how I feel. I want to be able to overcome my usual memory deficit and outline the symptoms to my physiatrist, whom I am going to see today. I have the usual tightness in my left arm and hand. Once again, my left arm feels like it is imbedded into my ribs so tightly that it is elbowing me to the point of seeming like it is penetrating my rib cage. I realize that it is a phantom sensation because I can actually lift my arm, which is reasonably loose right now and is not poking me at all. I am short of breath from the "supposed" force of the pressure and the outside of my index finger is stinging very intensely. I find I can wiggle my index finger and move my thumb up and down a little but as I observe them, I realize that they mostly just vibrate.

The very top of my scalp feels strained and is tingling as I concentrate and I feel a slight headache and numbness in my head as I sit at the computer trying to assemble my thoughts on the various sensations on the upper left side of my body. Of course, my leg is very stiff with a sharp tingling in my toes. I can't move my foot or toes at all and they hurt like hell. My head feels as though I have been scalped. When I am this uncomfortable, I sit here feeling as though I just want to lose consciousness and go to sleep and just forget everything that has happened to me. My eyes feel as though they are crossed or rolled up inside my head, a feeling I often have.

August 20, 2005

My family doctor sent me to a urologist the other day to attempt to discover why I was continually getting these bladder infections. We had decided that this was ridiculous and that enough was enough. Of course, every time I was feeling this lousy, I had learned that there was a recurring pattern and if I had finished a script of antibiotics for the previous bladder infection, I could almost be sure that I would soon be experiencing yet another urinary tract infection.

Did I ever tell you why I was so prone to bladder infections? It is actually due to the paralysis I have on my left side, a direct result of my stroke. It seems that a person in my situation does not necessarily empty his bladder quite as completely as one should during a pee. As a result, the likelihood of developing such an infection is higher than normal.

Well, during my visit with the urologist, he reviewed with Hélène and me the precise procedure that we were following when providing the sample. He almost immediately identified the problem. It seemed that we were taking the sample improperly and we didn't realize it. Whenever I would provide a urine sample, I would simply pee into the urinal beside the bed, like I always did each night. Afterwards, Hélène would pour the urine into the doctor's specimen bottle and drop it off for testing at the lab. This process had always gone fairly routinely. We would then bring the sample over to my doctor's office or to the local lab for analysis and usually within 48 hours our family physician would call us back and announce that, yes, I had another bladder infection!

Well, the urologist identified that we should not be transferring the urine from the urinal to the specimen bottle as the opportunity for developing bacteria was too great and so it was likely that the test would *always* indicate a bladder infection. Well not being medical experts, I guess there was no way that we would know this. Honestly, this problem never even occurred to us and it was not obvious to our family doctor because, of course, he was not at our house each time to actually witness and oversee the procedure. Well, talk about mind over matter! Once we had established the proper procedure and I was just peeing directly into the specimen bottle, we were no longer getting indications from the lab of positive test results and I guess I was no longer imagining I was getting a urinary tract infection. I have to honestly say that I have not had any further problem since we got the routine down pat. Mission successful! A nightmare is now behind me and I owe many thanks to my family physician and to my urologist for being so thorough and attentive.

And so it seems that Thalamic Pain is at the root of my discomfort.

August 31, 2005

So now I feel I will no longer be writing about these bladder infections as I don't seem to be suffering any of these miserable symptoms any more since working out the testing procedure. But this in no way is suggesting I am feeling great each day! I am still in excruciating pain (Thalamic Pain, I suppose) almost every day. My toes feel as though they are frostbitten and I feel a tingling through the length of my paralyzed left leg. Also, my left hand is usually quite sore, mostly along the length of my index and middle fingers. I feel as if I am receiving 1,000 bee stings and this pain lasts all day with no relief. To be honest, I am actually almost used to these sensations by now but they are painful and usually do seem to last all day. At least I seem to have eliminated the likelihood of discomfort from the UTIs. The remaining pain and discomfort is simply the Regional or Thalamic pain that I am enduring as a direct result of the paralysis throughout my left side.

September 2, 2005

Hélène and I are having an interesting morning. We woke up together at about 8:00 am. Hélène got up and went into the kitchen to make us some coffee. As usual, we had a project in mind and Hélène unpacked the lawn chair I bought her yesterday for our anniversary, which is coming up at the end of the month. She had bought me a new tennis racquet which was particularly special and with which I am very pleased. I opened the packing that contained the screws and lock washers. We lined up the parts according to the instructional diagram and began to slowly tighten each screw in sequence so that the chair slowly came together.

Unfortunately, as I may have explained elsewhere in my book, whenever I am concentrating or even simply figuring something out, such as reading instructions and assembling something as simple as a lawn chair, the long term effects of my brain surgery cause my head to buzz like crazy, making me very dizzy and longing for the relief that will give me a peaceful and calmer stability in my head. Let me tell you, I have had to learn to just grin and bear it. The buzzing is very intense and it crawls through my arm and leg and causes the bee-buzz in my head and the stinging effect in my hand, toes and fingers.

This feeling is not at all amusing. It is very intense and is almost unbearable. There is an acute ringing in my ear that just won't stop. I feel as though something is about to explode. I can just imagine my skull splitting open and brain matter splattering all over the room. Fortunately, it won't ever be quite that bad.

September 4, 2005

Hélène and I went to the tennis courts by our house today and hit tennis balls for about an hour. While I can rally reasonably well, it can be frustrating for me because I have to use only my right arm to swing the racquet and control my chair. I cannot move sideways quickly to the left or right with my chair, so my opponent has to be able to hit the ball close to me in order for me to be able to return it. I have a half-decent forehand and backhand, however.

Afterwards, we were talking to our neighbour, Dave, who offered to repair a leaky faucet at the side of our house. After inspecting it closely, Dave told us we needed a new faucet and so we drove to Home Depot to purchase the necessary part. When we came back, we went over to Dave and Heather's for a few drinks and some laughs. Even though my head isn't feeling the best, it's always good to spend time with nice people. I think we will probably have a quiet night together tonight. Maybe we'll watch a movie.

September 5, 2005

It is September 5th and I have now been recovering from my stroke for about two and a half years. As part of my recovery efforts, I have been taking physiotherapy for about 23 months and I have been working on this book for about six months.

Considering my brain damage, this book has been incredible mental therapy and I am simply having so much fun writing it. It is just like a vivid dream where everything I have been writing about seems like I have just relived it and I am enjoying growing up all over again.

Today is a gorgeous day. With no exaggeration, we have been enjoying the best summer I can recall. Every day since June 1st has been hot and sunny. Today, my personal trainer, Angie has been here to work with me, assisting me in flexing my muscles, bending my joints and generally overseeing my swimming for as many as 16 lengths. The swimming makes me feel so relaxed and relieves the ongoing spasticity and muscle tone.

Just before Angie came by, Hélène, Corey and I went to the driving range to hit a couple of buckets of golf balls. We usually get out a couple of times a week to hit at least two buckets between us. I am so delighted that my determination has enabled me to continue enjoying this sport, despite my left-side paralysis and resultant disability.

I am sitting out with Hélène on the deck of our pool in the backyard, enjoying a nice cool glass of Sangria under the warmth of a hot and sunny day. As I said, this summer has been magical and has been so good for me both mentally and physically. I am not looking forward to the winter and the cold but we are enjoying each hot summer day as it happens. Having a drink or two or the occasional glass of wine never seems to affect me or make me feel worse, but I do watch the amount I drink so that the alcohol does not suppress the benefit of any of the medication that I have taken on any particular day.

Since my stroke, I have been faithfully logging "how I feel" almost every day, because the pain and discomfort have been so unbearable that I just feel compelled to try to share my affliction with others, so that they can hopefully understand it.

As I sit at the patio table writing this piece, my head is experiencing its usual dizziness. As well, my toes are intensely painful, similar to the sensation of frostbite. Why does this happen? It's friggin' well 28º C outside so it can't be actual frostbite! I am forced to accept that this is a seeming "phantom" sensation as a result of my brain damage and resulting surgery. I have been reading that this is Thalamic or Regional pain. The internet is a tremendous resource and I have been looking everything up. My left leg and arm as well as the left side of my face are numb but, fortunately, the physical features on my face are not affected. Most people say that I am looking great, considering how terrible I looked when I first went into the hospital. My head has extreme pressure, making it difficult to concentrate and causing the occasional tear of pain to fall down my cheek. Yes, I can be a whiner.

This afternoon, I am trying to concentrate on writing a few paragraphs for my book and I am planning to have

Hélène wheel me back into the house through the patio door in Corey's room to get into our bedroom and change from my damp swimsuit into some dry clothes. I am anxious to get my shoes and socks on to cover up and help relieve the stinging in my toes. My toes are now very sensitive. I have had a good day, but I have had enough of the outdoors. I need a change of scenery.

September 7, 2005

It is now almost three weeks since I have had any indication of a bladder infection. This is very bizarre but, for some reason, I am no longer experiencing even the tiniest discomfort from a possible urinary tract infection. Who knows? Maybe each time I was just talking myself into believing I was being overcome with the infection when, in reality, it was just a case of mind over matter! I am so relieved to no longer be affected by this discomfort.

December 1, 2005

Ironically, after all my whining and complaining about "how I feel" overall, I am starting to feel much better. I do not quite feel great by any means but I have not been getting bladder infections nor have I been receiving positive urine tests when I submit them to the doctor's office.

It has actually been about three months since I have written down any of these discomforts. I guess I might even say that I am just getting too damn used to the pain, inconvenience and all of the discomfort that goes with having to live with having had a stroke.

The good news is that, despite the fact that I am still a good distance from a full recovery and back to normal functionality, I am enjoying life with my boys and my wife and Cooper, our amazing Golden Retriever. Also, despite many of my earlier logs about the hell I had been going through with bladder infections, I am somehow now getting by on a day-to-day basis without having any indication of any bladder infections. This is very bizarre but, for some reason, I simply am no longer experiencing what had become a routine nightmare for me. My family physician and Urologist discovered that I had not been following a recommended procedure for providing urine tests so my tests were invalid, usually indicating an infection was present when there wasn't any. Also my family physician prescribed the appropriate medication and encouraged me to drink lots of fluids including cranberry juice. The amusing thing was that I seemed to be convincing myself that I was repeatedly getting UTIs. It was all psychological, I guess.

So, with these episodes apparently behind me, I have proceeded with Taoist Tai Chi at the local club right here in my home town, and I am now also seeing an acupuncturist who treats me twice a week. I also take Chinese (herbal) medicine twice a day. Do I really know if these treatments are helping me? No, not really. I just know that my family physician supports it and he and others actually truly believe in it. Also, I am told that, because the prepared herbal medicine is such a mild dose, it will take a long time to produce results. At this point, considering my condition, can I truly afford not to try these methods? I personally don't think so. The relief and potential recovery is priceless.

December 5, 2005

Guess what? Still no further bladder infections! Something has stabilized. Thank goodness.

December 29, 2005

Today, as is my new and now, current routine, Hélène drove me downtown to Chinatown where I see my acupuncturist twice a week. This experienced gentleman has been working in Toronto for seven years and has been practicing acupuncture for a total of 46 years. Prior to immigrating to Canada, he was the head acupuncturist at one of China's largest hospitals. Our drive from home is almost one hour each way down the Don Valley Parkway, usually right around rush hour, and Hélène usually loses me to a solid power snooze for most of the drive. I usually wake up just as we are arriving at the doctor's office and Hélène helps me out of the van and transfers me into my chair where I wait for her to park the van. She then comes back and escorts me on my ride in the elevator up to the 5th floor. As we get off the elevator, she guides me down the immense, long hallway of the apartment building to the doctor's suite. The doctor has been encouraging me to walk with a new walker since I have been seeing him and I must say I have achieved a noticeable improvement with it.

Initially, I experienced extreme pain whenever I held on to anything with my left hand. I can now truly say I am able to grip the walker with little or no difficulty. I enter his treatment room and lie on my right side, exposing my left side and he uncovers the treatment areas where he will insert the acupuncture needles. He usually places about seven or eight tiny acupuncture needles down my left side and along my shoulder, arm and wrist as well as my hip, knee, and ankle. Also, lately, I have been complaining about some considerable pain in my fingers and toes (Thalamic Pain, I believe) so he has increased the number of needles he inserts into my hand and foot. In fact today, I was complaining about pain across my face, ear and neck so he administered some needles to my face as well. Initially, the thought of this was a little unnerving; but I never really felt the needles going in and the result was a sense of relief and a numbing of the stinging pain I had felt prior to the session. As I lay half asleep on his treatment bed, the doctor started his systematic routine of inserting about eight or more needles. I closed my eyes and nearly drifted off as I barely sensed the occasional pin prick. I can honestly say that I usually undergo the entire procedure without feeling a single prick. Once in a while, I have looked over at a particular insertion and noticed that, after placing the needle in the appropriate place by tapping it home, he has occasionally twisted and pushed the needle deeper, likely to achieve the effective penetration for the particular area being treated.

On the way home and into the evening, I have to say that the pain in my hand and foot was barely noticeable, thank God!

Now, if I wanted to I could write a lengthy piece again about the experiences and benefits of Taoist Tai Chi. Rather than do that, I will refer you to Section Eight, Chapter 2.

January 23, 2006

I have just woken from a sound and peaceful sleep. Unfortunately, Hélène woke up a lot overnight and is quite tired this morning. My darling wife is downstairs, making our breakfast which, in my case this morning, will include a lightly toasted bagel with raspberry jam and of course my Chinese medicine. As I was sitting in my wheelchair, typing away at my PC, I was adding this piece to my book. I lay in bed part of the night, with my mind once more racing with many thoughts and ideas for my book. Whenever I do this, my head plays tricks on me and my mind gets cluttered with so many new ideas (the traffic thing) that I simply tell myself I have to get creative and download them to my book file.

Last night was an incredible experience. I was feeling the relatively typical CPS (Complex Central Pain Syndrome or Thalamic Pain). These experiences are quite intense and very uncomfortable. When it is occurring, my toes and fingers feel as though they have been stung by a hive of bees, my joints ache and my skin hurts. So tonight I took a couple of tablets of Lyrica, a new wonder drug my family physician prescribed for me. Thank God, it always seems to relieve my discomfort!

February 15, 2006

This is how I was feeling this afternoon before I had my prescription and my Chinese medicine:

Very lethargic;
Very dizzy;
Pain and tightness in my face and lips;
Slurred speech;
Pain in my right knee;
Pain in my left foot (severe Achilles tendon pain); and,
Pain in the toes of my left foot.

After taking both my pain medication and my Chinese medicine and putting ice on it, my knee felt better and mostly I just felt the tightness and discomfort of the pressure in my head.

The pain in my Achilles tendon was a little better and I was still a bit lethargic, but not quite as much as I was earlier.

February 20, 2006

I woke up at 4:00 am today and decided to haul myself out of bed, get into my wheelchair and go into the computer room and work a little on my book, which is making good progress. I feel (hope) that I am only less than a month away from actually sending my manuscript to the publisher. The writing process so far has been an incredibly interesting journey, detailing so many aspects of my life and my nightmare. I often tell myself that, even if I never actually get this book published, the entire process will have been worth it, if only for its neurological therapeutic value/benefit.

I have not been feeling the best over the past couple of days, feeling extremely stiff and spastic on my left side. Of course, so far, since having my stroke, my left leg and arm are always painfully stiff as a board but these past few days, my whole left side is tingly, numb and sore. The skin on the left side of my face feels tight, my lower lip is numb and my leg and arm are excessively stiff. My scheduled caregiver, Leanne, gave me a shower this morning and I was initially very uncomfortable getting onto my transfer bench and finally into the shower and under the warm water, which, I have to admit, was so relaxing.

So, at the moment, I am sitting at my computer, reflecting on all my feelings, sensations and pains, as I do most days. I do so want to take a pill or have something surgically removed so that I feel better. I am taking a new prescription for pain at the current time, called Lyrica, that usually helps me feel better but honestly, I enjoy and appreciate my acupuncture treatments the most. They bring me so much relief. At this moment, my fingers and toes feel like they are being stung by 1,000 angry bees. The left side of my rib cage feels like my left elbow is pressing into it at considerable force, although, in reality, it isn't. My skin feels tight, as though it is three or four sizes too small for my actual torso and my fingers are curled and stiff, although not curled as tightly or completely clenched as they used to be.

Today, in addition to all my usual stroke-related discomfort, I seem to have slightly sprained my *right* thumb, wrist and palm. I have some pain around the knuckle between my *right* thumb and wrist. It appears that I have probably sprained these when lifting myself out of or into bed or from or into my wheelchair. I don't remember exactly doing it at all. I just know it hurts so I had Leanne rub on some "Polar Ice", analgesic gel to relieve it. I also am icing it as I speak. I have decided to miss my Taoist Tai Chi class today because I was so uncomfortable with these extra aches and pains. If it wasn't for them, I would have gone to my Tai Chi class because I enjoy it and because it is so good for rebuilding my strength and mobility.

March 10, 2006

Today is Friday, March 10, 2006 and I am not feeling very good, especially in my head. My entire head and body are tingling, actually sort of like vibrating. The sensation in my head is as if an electric current was running through it. I am experiencing a tingling (like burning) on my right leg and the hair follicles on both legs hurt and feel like they are burning as they rub on the bed sheets. Also, my left leg aches. My left arm and hand tingle (like they are being stung). The left side of my head hurts (my ear and my face). I am also a little out of breath, even though I am lying down watching television. But I guess I am actually getting used to this pain and discomfort.

Excuse me while I whine a little. I have left side paralysis which means I have no use of my left side. For months since being released from my rehabilitation program at Bridgepoint Health, I have been pursuing numerous recovery efforts to hopefully regain some reasonable use of my left arm and leg. It is a long, slow haul with no promises or guarantees. The most promise I have seen has been from doing many Don Yus in my Taoist Tai Chi classes and, of course, at home as I practice.

At this time, I am in the process of trying to figure out exactly how I want to finish my book. I am researching and trying to find someone who will be interested in publishing this project; I am not certain exactly how to proceed from here but Hélène and I have drawn out a couple of books from the local library that will hopefully point us in the right direction.

As I write my story and work so very hard to complete my book, my dear friends, family and loved ones, I wish to state to you, right now, that I am 53 years old and I can't believe that I have been writing about my life going as far back as when I was only 5 years old and actually remembering those days as if they had happened within the past few weeks. To think that in seven years I will be 60 years old! I still think, dream and recall events as though I was only 28 or 29 years old. I guess it's kind of immature, isn't it? But who cares? I am a seriously sick man with a confused mind and the only thing that is important is that I enjoy myself and that I love those that love and care about me. Gees, I feel like crap today.

I want this book to be helpful to other stroke survivors. I hope I am doing a good job of reaching this objective. I am certainly no expert or experienced writer but I am currently thinking about how to finish this book and of some of the ideas that I can incorporate into my next book which I have already started. I think my new book will be a science fiction with some adventure, murder and mystery. I hope you enjoy it. I hope it is not confusing. I hope you have enjoyed this book. I hope it benefits others. That's all that matters.

So guess what? Read back five paragraphs and read where I was telling you how poorly I was feeling today. Well, I am actually feeling a bit better at this moment. I only have a stinging in my fingers, mostly my left thumb and index finger but my head is rather thick and buzzy and I am quite dizzy. I thought I was never going to feel better.

March 25, 2006

Actually, tomorrow happens to be my birthday. A few friends are coming over this evening to enjoy some wine and a few laughs, just a last minute thing with a few neighbours.

Hélène and I got up and were out of the house fairly early this morning. I had an appointment to go up the street to the local lab to get a blood test done for my cholesterol; no big deal, just a routine follow-up test for my family doctor after visiting him earlier this week. I am particularly interested in my cholesterol levels because, with my paralysis, I am apt to be less active and get less exercise overall, so it is desirable that I keep them within acceptable levels so that I can enjoy a wider range of my favourite foods. Other than the other obvious issues from my stroke, I am in excellent health. Yes, I do whine and complain a bit about the pain and dizziness, as well as the tightness and spasticity from the effects of the paralysis and the brain surgery and all that. However, I am fortunate that my doctor has discovered no medical issues otherwise. In fact, my weight is optimum, my appetite is excellent and my bowels and plumbing are working just fine.

This week was another week of miracles. After not having been able to walk since my stroke back in February, 2003, I actually took a few steps unassisted the other day from my specially equipped passenger seat in our van to the side door. I opened it to get a book from the back seat. I am now wearing a brace made for my left leg and foot which is working amazingly well. The brace was made by Mike, an orthotist at the nearby "Ortho-Tek". Mike is another one of those amazing "magical" people whom I am frequently encountering throughout this nightmare experience. These special people I am fortunate enough to be encountering all seem to be providing such excellent service and are able and want to find appropriate solutions to some of my problems. By the way, Mike, it seems that some of your colleagues over at the Whitby Day Hospital are suitably impressed by your skills and professionalism, as well. Another 10 from Peter's

1 to 10 Customer Service Rating System goes out to Mike. Thanks, Mike!

March 28, 2006

Today, for some unexplained reason, I feel outstanding. I have no pain, no real discomfort and physically I actually feel as though I could just stride across the room. I'm not about to kid myself, however. I have cautiously tested my leg and arm and they are definitely still paralyzed. It's just that I feel great. I actually don't quite believe I can be feeling this good. Mind you, my head is not totally relaxed and calm. But there is no pressure today and I am quite relaxed and comfortable. I have to stop and reflect on each of my nerve endings and on my limbs. For whatever reason, they are feeling very comfortable. This is highly unusual. I am wondering what neurological circumstance is causing this to happen.

Yesterday, Hélène and I drove three and a half hours to get to Renfrew to visit my Dad. We visited for about three hours and had a pleasant "catch up" time, enjoying a meal of KFC that we picked up just on the edge of town. Our niece, Megan, ate with us while her Mom (my sister) had to go to a union meeting at work. I did not feel the best. In fact, I felt my usual self, stricken with Thalamic Pain and feeling thick-headed and a little lethargic. Nothing unusual there.

April 13, 2006

Today was a particularly bad day. My head was terribly uncomfortable. I didn't have a headache so Tylenol wasn't about to be a solution. In fact, there is no direct medication for what I feel in my head when I get this way. All I can do is try to take it slow and just bear it. My head feels as though a pair of women's pantyhose has been pulled over it and the legs tightly knotted so that I cannot breakout or let my skin breathe. I am incredibly dizzy so my vision is slightly blurred and my eyelids twitch so I cannot see clearly. I cannot think straight and I would like to go for a nap. Of course, my toes and fingers sting and I yawn a lot. The fingers on my left hand clench and the backs of my fingers feel immense pressure. The soles of my feet hurt.

Oh yes, did I mention that I am walking with my cane a lot? I had been getting around for the past year or so in my power wheelchair when outside or traveling around the mall or playing wheelchair tennis but I wheel myself around the house in my manual chair. In fact, Hélène and I did go out to the pub for a beer, some soup and a salad tonight but it felt good to wind up the evening and go home and get into bed.

This has been the norm for the past two years, but in the past few weeks I have been getting up and walking around the house and the front walk and down the hallways of certain buildings and such with my cane. It has all been quite miraculous actually. I was beginning to think that I would never get to this point in my recovery; but thanks to Tai Chi, my physiotherapists and my own perseverance, I have been walking at every opportunity and getting stronger as I go. I do still need to regain some use of my left arm so that I can hold my balance and grip things.

April 19, 2006

Today was a much better day than yesterday. My head was a lot clearer, calmer and much more stable. As well,

I did not have much of the anxious feeling I usually get deep down inside. I still have the tightness I usually feel in my face, due to the paralysis. My head is a little tight still. I have had a lot of energy today and was walking everywhere. I even walked outside to the very back corner of our back yard and perched myself on a stump with an axe Hélène borrowed from a neighbour and I hacked away some fungus that had been growing on the stump. Hélène and I were working together at some very aggressive yard spring cleaning.

The fingers on my left hand though are firmly clenched and the backs of my fingers feel tingly and feel like many bee stings. Also, the soles of my feet and my toes hurt. Some things just don't change!

April 20, 2006

I have woken up today, feeling pretty much as I did yesterday. I am actually not used to getting up and feeling OK. I certainly do still have the usual discomforts such as the stinging fingers and toes, the numb lips and minor head buzzing but I think I will probably be reasonably comfortable today.

May 20, 2006

On Monday, the 8th I was feeling kind of lousy, pretty much the same as I had been feeling for most of the last few months. I had lots of Thalamic Pain, a shortness of breath and my fingers and toes hurt (like frostbite, as usual).

I had been experiencing extreme pain in the past few weeks and had an appointment to see my neurologist on

Thursday, May 11th. Unfortunately, his office called to reschedule my appointment to a week later, so Hélène made an appointment for me with my family doctor on Wednesday, the 10th. I saw him and he prescribed Elavil for the pain and it seems to be helping. I am still concerned about the reason and the source of this discomfort. I saw my physiatrist on the following Monday, May 15th. He said that my pain is probably from the thalamus in my brain and he prescribed a CT scan as an update and to verify that no metal was left in my brain during surgery which could be dangerous as metal left inside could create problems with an MRI. The request has been faxed to the hospital and a scan has now been scheduled for May 30th.

I seemed to be feeling a little better by the following Thursday, so I foolishly rescheduled my appointment with my neurologist. Later that day, I was suddenly not exactly sure how good I was going to be feeling so I started to think I made a mistake by cancelling the appointment.

Throughout the day on Friday, I think I was feeling much better. I ended up having a pretty good day. Then Friday night at around 10:00 pm, Brian called us to talk to us about Dad. He said it was possible Dad had had a small stroke. I started to feel very bad. I was developing the familiar pain in my toes and fingers with a shortness of breath and pain in my face and teeth. My brain was not handling this news and the overall traffic very well. The thalamic pain was back. I must have fallen asleep around 1:00 am, after watching a couple of episodes of CSI.

I slept like a baby that night with Hélène and me waking up at only 10:30 am, what a treat!

The following is a letter that I sent to my neurologist a couple of days later:

"Dear Dr. XXXX,

This letter is further and in addition to my letter of May 18.

For the last few weeks or more, I have been experiencing intense, ongoing complex thalamic pain to my extremities on the left side and my head is undergoing intense pressure and dizziness. I just can't find any calm or relaxation where my head and left side of my body do not have a terrible and unrelenting pain.

This pain and discomfort does not subside. Should I go to a hospital?

As I am writing this, I am feeling the sensation of cool air blowing against my arms, my upper body (chest) and my face, including my nostrils. It feels like I am in sub-zero temperature or driving a car in below zero temperature with the windows down and my head out of the window. Covering my face under the bed covers does not seem to make this sensation stop at the time but most of it is gone when I wake up the next morning although I continue to feel a cool wind (like a breeze) against my face. Is this what I understand to be *complex central or thalamic pain*? Can any thing be done to treat or relieve it?

I originally had an appointment to see you on May 11 but your office unfortunately called and postponed it to May 18 which I regrettably had to miss for another appointment. I also had an appointment with and did see my physiatrist on May 15 as a follow up to my last Botox injections. He ordered a CT Scan to update and compare against my last CT Scan. The doctor felt that a CT Scan would be more helpful at this time to determine that no metal had been left in my head during my surgery in 2003 which apparently could be harmful if an MRI were performed to investigate the source of this discomfort.

I did not get a response or comment from you in reply to my letter of May 18 and I am now scheduled to see you on July 19. Please tell me what we can do or what I can expect.

Thank you.

Peter"

June 18, 2006

Well, now it is June 18th and we have had a pretty good start to the summer. We have just had our pool opened and are anxious to start using it. Of course, we appreciate the pool heater as it makes the water so much more pleasant and so much more bearable for me. I need to have it at about 95ºF since my stroke. Any cooler and I just find it too uncomfortable. It actually hurts and causes me to stiffen up.

Unfortunately, we have been struggling with the heater and its pilot light. Dave F. has been over religiously a few times to reset it. We have been made aware that the law prohibits the staff from the pool supply store with which we deal from lighting the pilot light. It can only be lit by a licensed gas contractor. So, until we get the heater reliably lit, repaired or stable, we unfortunately constantly bug Dave. However, he always seems to be there and comes through for us. Geez, Dave, thanks so much. I guess the good part is that it just ends up being another excuse to enjoy his and Heather's company over a few beers!

July 11, 2006

It's interesting that I mention a couple of major milestones here. You will have previously observed a series of entries in this "How I Feel" section, where I spoke about a seemingly unrelenting pattern of recurring UTIs (urinary tract infections). You will also note that on August 20 of last year (2005), I reported that a urologist I had an appointment with had determined that we were unknowingly collecting my urine samples in a contaminated bottle, thus consistently resulting in continuous positive test results.

Once the correct procedure had been established, the UTIs ceased and I am happy to say that they are no longer happening at all.

Another rather exciting moment (well, exciting for Hélène and me anyway) was when I actually started swimming without a life jacket, for the first time since my stroke, on July 1 of this year. Don't get me wrong, I wasn't quite ready to do a complete proper front crawl, but I was able to pull myself through the water for a few laps with my one good arm. I had been kicking nicely with both legs since early last year.

Also, I need to mention here that, while I still incur considerable pain on a daily basis, it has been determined that the primary cause of my discomfort is thalamic pain, a syndrome that usually afflicts stroke victims about a year or so after their initial brain attack. Based on what I have read, it is possible that such pain will continue indefinitely.

SPECIAL ACKNOWLEDGEMENTS

I wish to express my heartfelt thanks and appreciation to the following people/groups for supporting and encouraging me in this effort, as well as their knowledge and permission to share information and use it in this book:

- Expert Tree Service: Tree Service and Stump Grinding
  905-666-0063 (Steve)
- Falkirk Construction Group: Fencing, Renovations, Carpentry, Landscape Design, Handyman Services & General Construction
  905-925-6294 (Adrian)
- Garden Design by Beata
  905-665-6294 (Beata)
- Home Depot – Ajax
  905-428-7939 (Eamon)
- Medichair Durham
  905-666-5001 (Ray)
- International Taoist Tai Chi Society
  Health Recovery Centre
  519-941-7991 (Mary, Kelly and Bernice)
- International Taoist Tai Chi Society Head Office,
  www.taoist.org
  416-656-2110
- Heart & Stroke Foundation of Ontario
  905-666-3777
- Lakeridge Health Whitby – Whitby Day Hospital
  905-668-6831

- Nice-Bistro
    905-668-8839 (Bernard et Manon)
- Krebs Restaurant
    905-668-9369 (Gary and Patricia)
- Avalon Dental Care
    905-665-2353 (Mark & staff)
- Points & Needles Acupuncture Clinic
    905-430-0137 (Erik)
- StrokeSafe.org
- Central Pain Syndrome Alliance, www.centralpain.org
- Wikipedia, the Free Encyclopedia, www.wikipedia.org
- American Academy of Family Physicians, www.aafp.org
- Variety Village, www.varietyontario.ca
- Ontario Wheelchair Sports,
    www.ontwheelchairsports.org
- Angus Glen Golf Club, www.angusglen.com
- ebay, www.ebay.com
- Bridgepoint Health, www.bridgepointhealth.ca
- Head Injury Association of Durham Region,
    www.durham.cioc.ca
- Stroke Recovery Systems, www.neuromove.com

Printed in the United States
66503LVS00003B/4-24